I0493321

This protocol is for informational purposes only. It has NOT been evaluated by the FDA, nor is it intended to treat any disease, illness or sickness.

It is designed to educate the reader on many of the current mechanical therapies and nutritional therapies available, which MAY accelerate the rate at which the body heals.

Every person who reads this is totally in charge of their own health…and their own healing. You (and your medical professional) are totally responsible for implementing any procedures found within this protocol.

The Rapid Bone Repair Protocol™

The Rapid Bone Repair Protocol™ (The Full Monty)

I. Introduction

If you are reading this protocol either you or a loved one probably has "broken" or "fractured" a bone. This introduction to the physiology of how bones are repaired by your body and to the nutritional and physical needs that a "bone repair" requires should help you to understand how the "healing" process will eventually occur (Naturally), and how we can significantly "speed up" that repair process by following these best practices. This report will cite many medical studies, but will not be "clinical" or "technical" in nature. I will try to use common language so the protocol is easily understood. Cited studies can be found at the end of the protocol for more detailed study (for those who are interested).

These steps are not "magic bullets" nor are they a "miracle cure." The amount of time that your fracture will take to heal depends on many factors specific to your (and only your) injury. These factors include, but are not limited to:

- The severity of the fracture (the number of broken bones, the extent of the damage),
- The type of fracture,
- Is the fracture sticking through the skin?
- Is there potential infection at the site?
- Is this a repeat injury?
- Are there other injuries alongside the fracture? (Ligaments, tendons, soft tissue organs)

- Your general state of health when the injury occurred,
- Your allergies & health issues,
- Your age,
- The general health of your immune system

The one thing that all of these have in common is that they are OUT OF YOUR CONTROL. You can't go back in time and prepare yourself better for the fracture. Since the fracture has already occurred, we will be focusing on tangible physical and nutritional steps that you can take FROM HERE ON OUT that will allow your body to heal as quickly as possible.

ALL of the steps in the Rapid Bone Repair Protocol are IN YOUR CONTROL. You do not need to simply sit back and wait passively for your body to eventually get the job done. Your body is amazing, and can repair itself from dramatic trauma. But, why not help it along? Why not stack the cards in your favor, so that you can reduce the "recuperative" time, and quickly get back to your "normal" activities?

Your body will eventually get the job done without your input at all (in most cases). Your body will self-immobilize the fracture, and will leech the needed minerals for the repair from your other bones (depleting them in the process), and you will eventually get back on your feet. But, why sit back passively and make it difficult for your body to heal itself? We now understand how the body goes about healing fractures, and with this medical and scientific knowledge, along with some common sense, we can help the healing process along.... Rather than simply being passive observers.

If you are a professional athlete or a worker or a parent, time on the sidelines is money. Getting back in the game, as quickly as possible, is important, if not absolutely necessary. We cannot stay on the sideline for long, certainly for no longer than we absolutely HAVE TO. This protocol is perfect for you!

This protocol has personally worked for me multiple times. As a competitive athlete, I was not willing to "sit it out", but was motivated to help my body heal as quickly as possible. If you are interested, you can read my story, dealing with the first versions of this protocol in the appendix. That being said, your injury is specific to you. You and your healthcare practitioner are the ones who need to examine the evidence presented, and decide on your course of action. This protocol works, and it is currently being used by doctors, chiropractors, physical therapists and other healthcare professionals, but YOU and YOUR healthcare professional will need to supervise YOUR specific recovery plan. In other words, this protocol does not give you the ability to simply bypass your health provider, but it should be monitored by your healthcare provider. This protocol is informational and educational, but your custom treatment plan should be prescribed by your healthcare provider (in light of the recommendations made in this protocol).

The "healing arts" have been going on for thousands of years. We should learn from our ancestors and potentially take some of their accumulated wisdom and apply it today. This protocol therefore, looks at some ancient medicinal advice, but combines that with the latest scientific, nutritional and medical studies available. This protocol truly takes the best of both worlds and synthesizes them together to give your body the very best "treatment" options available.

The protocol is divided into sections. The first section will give a general overview of normal healthy bones and then the types of fractures, and how the body normally repairs a fractured bone. In this section, we will define certain terms, and we can see physiologically what occurs from the time of fracture, up until the time when the bone can be considered "repaired." After this introductory chapter, we will jump right in to the "Bone Repair Protocol" and look at the physical recommendations (the first three protocols). These are physical and mechanical things that you can do to speed up the bone healing process. The next 4 steps in the protocol all deal with nutritional recommendations that you should follow to fuel your body with the necessary "stuff" to rapidly get back in the game. Following the Protocol, we have a chapter quickly dealing with long term bone health… and how this protocol can be modified to work well on a permanent basis to continually keep your bones as healthy as possible.

II. Bones and Bone Fractures

Bone is a living tissue

It is easy to think that our bones are made up of lifeless matter, which gives structure to our skeletal system. But your skeleton is very much a living part of your body - similar to your softer tissues and organs. Your body stores minerals in the hard, compact bone. The bone produces red blood cells in the inner red marrow, and it stores fat in the yellow marrow.

Your bones are useful for the structure of your body (for support, for leverage, for protection, etc.), but they are also important as storage centers (minerals and fat) and as actual blood factories.

It is also true that your bones are constantly remaking themselves. This process of "remodeling" takes place when cells called osteoclasts break down the old bone (deconstruction/demolition), so that osteoblasts (re-construction/new construction) can replace it with new bone tissue. Two different types of cells called a chondroblast and a fibroblast (re)form and produce new cartilage. These four types of cells are the primary cells responsible for bone removal and new bone growth.

This constant remodeling of the bones does not just occur as a child, and then stop as an adult. No- there is constant bone remodeling that gradually replaces old bone tissue with new bone tissue. This remodeling process only stops at death. Until then, your body will be constantly "renovating" the bones in your skeletal system. Your body remodels between 2% and 4% of your skeletal system each year.

Types of Fractures

There are many types of fractures. In a complete fracture, the bone snaps into two or more separate parts. An incomplete fracture consists of some type of a crack or splintering, but the parts of the bone are still connected - the break does not go all the way through the bone making separate parts.

In a compound fracture, also called an open fracture, the bone breaks through the skin; it may then recede back into the wound, and not be visible through the skin. This type of fracture carries with it an increased risk of infection - due to the skin barrier being damaged, and potentially allowing bacteria, dirt, and possibly other matter into the wound.

In a simple fracture, also called a closed fracture, the bone breaks (either completely or incompletely), but there is no open wound through the skin.

Simple fractures include:

- Greenstick fracture: an incomplete fracture, in which the bone is bent, and half of it is splintered, like a green tree limb. This type occurs most often in children.
- Transverse fracture: a fracture at a right angle to the bone's axis. This occurs often in the long bones of the arms and legs.

- An impacted fracture is one whose ends are driven into each other.
- A pathological fracture is caused by a disease that weakens the bones, until they fracture from some (possibly slight) trauma.
- A stress fracture is normally a hairline crack that occurs from a single trauma or, more commonly, from repeated trauma (such as of a long distance runner).
- A double fracture is where two or more bones are broken simultaneously.
- A spiral fracture is a corkscrew-like damage to the bone (very unstable).
- An oblique fracture is where the bone is broken at an angle.
- A compression fracture is where a bone has been crushed (normally from a fall or something similar).
- A comminuted bone fracture is where two or more parts of a bone have broken off from the same section of bone (it is very unstable).

These fracture categories are simply an introduction to all of the possible ways that bone can be damaged. Of course, there can also be multiple fractures, which mix and match different types of fractures. Each of these types of fracture is incredibly painful. Add that pain to a loss of mobility, and each fracture is extremely inconvenient.

Steps in the Bone Repair Process

Immediately after fracture has occurred, the body begins to repair the damage. Your body knows how to fix itself, and it is amazing to see the steps in the process of bone repair:

1. The Reactive Phase (Your body quickly reacts to the damage)

When the bone breaks, the blood vessels that are running the length of the bone break as well. Blood quickly leaks out of these veins, and forms a clot called a fracture hematoma. This hematoma (basically a collection or "clot" of blood outside of blood vessels) helps to stabilize the fractured ends of the bone, and keep them lined up for mending. The clot also cuts off the flow of blood to the jagged bone edges (to stop the internal bleeding). Without fresh blood, these bone cells on the very ends quickly die. Swelling and inflammation follow, due to the work of blood-cells starting to remove dead and damaged tissue. Tiny blood vessels grow into the fracture hematoma to fuel the healing process.

This fracture hematoma is the beginning of the re-connection of the pieces of bone. From this moment forward, this hematoma will begin to transform into firmer and firmer cells, providing more and more stability and strength, until the bone is completely "healed." During this repair process, if the hematoma, (or soft callus, or firbrocartilaginous callus) is re-separated by a further trauma, recovery will be slowed dramatically.

2. The Restorative Phase (Your body begins restoration)

After several days, the fracture hematoma (or "stabilizing blood clot") develops tougher tissue, transformed into a soft callus or "fracture callus." This callus gives stability to the bone ends as healing continues. Sometimes, this callus is referred to as a "cartilage scaffold."

Two types of cells quickly get to work to transform this soft callus into an even tougher and more stable connection. Fibroblasts begin producing fibers of collagen, the major protein in bone and connective tissue. Chondroblasts begin to produce a type of cartilage called fibrocartilage. These transform the soft callus into a tougher fibrocartilaginous callus, which strengthens and bridges the gap between the two pieces of bone.

Next, osteoblasts produce bone cells, slowly transforming the fibrocartilaginous callus into a bony callus. This harder callus provides necessary protection and stability for the bone to enter the final stage of healing. From this point on, the body will be constantly increasing the strength and rigidity of the type of bone in the callus.

The initial injury was stabilized as a blood clot, which then progressed to a soft callus composed primarily of collagen. The Callus then moves to fibrocartilage, then to woven bone, then on to lamellar bone, then on to trabecular bone. The body is incrementally and consistently strengthening and "improving" the strength of the callus, until the complete recovery of the bone.

3. The Re-Modeling Phase (Bone repair is finalized with "finishing touches")

The body establishes the "final" position of the bone within the flesh, begins reabsorbing bits of dead bone, and creates an even harder bone callus to bridge the gap between the two pieces of bone. The bone is almost as strong as before the fracture. Osteoclasts work to re-absorb the trabecular bone, and osteoblasts replace the trabecular bone with harder "compact bone". These cells also decrease the callus bulge, gradually returning the bone to its original shape.

We can see that the bone repair process is intricate, complex and absolutely amazing. To speed up this process, we simply need to understand what is happening at each step, and help our body with specific physical means (when needed) and nutritional means (also when needed) so that the body has all of the raw materials necessary, at the exact time it needs them.

III. The Bone Repair Protocol

The protocol has 3 physical recommendations, and 4 nutritional recommendations. We will initially look at the 3 Physical recommendations. These physical recommendations are ways that we can treat the broken bone, apart from our nutritional or food intake. It has to do with physical therapy, with protection of the fracture site, with attempting to increase the blood flow to the injured area…. In other words, these are steps that you can, and should, be taking that do not have to do with pills or chemicals or anything that you would ingest. These steps will not alter the chemical makeup of your body, but will still be very helpful in allowing your body to heal the fracture as quickly as possible.

A. Physical Recommendations

1.   Protocol ONE: Initially Immobilize and Protect the injured bone

Every fractured bone will need to be re-aligned to the correct anatomical position professionally, and as quickly as possible. This "reduction" or re-alignment is normally done with some type of traction or "pulling", which allows the fractured bone-ends to separate slightly, so that the bone can naturally re-align without too much grinding. This re-alignment is normally checked with an x-ray to make sure that it is lined up correctly. In some cases, the bones will not re-align with simple pulling, and continual traction may be necessary (temporarily). Or, in severe cases, the fracture may need to be opened up and re-aligned surgically (typically done with screws, wire, plates, rods, etc., in a very mechanical fashion).

If the re-alignment of the bone has not taken place correctly, it may be necessary (in some cases) to re-fracture the callus, which has formed at the fracture site, in order to correctly re-align the bone.

Once the fracture has been reduced, the fractured site should not be allowed to re-bend or be separated again. This normally is not an issue, because naturally your body will try to protect the fracture site. It hurts to "move" or "jar" the fractured bone, so our body naturally will "protect" any broken bone.

In order to keep the bones aligned and protected the doctors will try to immobilize and stabilize the bone in that correct alignment. They will try to come up with a way to allow the body to keep that fractured bone in alignment, while it heals. Normally, a cast is sufficient to accomplish this. A cast is like a temporary exo-skeleton, which allows your damaged endo-(inner)-skeleton to heal itself.

If a cast will not keep the bone aligned correctly, there may be other mechanical means of bone alignment, like straps, splints, "traction", belts - or other medieval-looking devices.

The blood clot that has formed at the fracture site should NOT be re-bent or re-broken, if at all possible, once the initial "reduction" has correctly repositioned the fractured bone. From the moment of the initial fracture, that blood clot will be working overtime to increasingly solidify, to strengthen, to become callus, and then to eventually become bone.

Protocol ONE is common practice in medical treatment of fractured bones. This step will probably already have been done by your healthcare provider by the time you are reading this protocol.

The main thing to remember here is not to re-fracture the blood clot/callus/cartilage/soft bone as it is in the healing process. There are three forces that should be protected against: shear, bending and twisting.

Shear happens when the two loose ends of the bone are kept pressing against each other, but one moves to the left, while the other moves to the right. It is a grinding of the bone-ends. You should not allow your fractured bones to shear against each

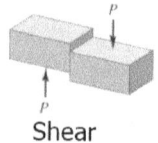

Shear

other. This will definitely slow the healing process. Now, normally a cast will give significant protection against shear forces.

Bending happens when the unbroken ends of the fracture are forced downward, while the fracture location itself is forced upwards (or vice versa). This force could easily damage the blood clot/callus, and the result is a longer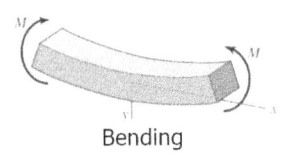

Bending

time required for healing. Fortunately, a regular cast also gives good protection from bending forces.

Twisting happens when one bone turns clockwise, while the other bone is turned counterclockwise. This type of a force on a callus or blood clot could cause the blood clot or callus to be damaged, resulting in slower healing of the fracture. Again, a normal "cast" will typically protect the fracture from twisting.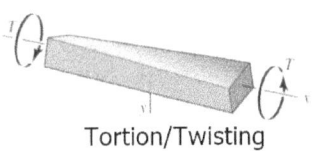

Tortion/Twisting

So Protocol One is to initially immobilize and protect the fracture site. Seems like a "no brainer." There is some medical evidence however, that **minor** movement of the "repairing" bone is actually beneficial. Because of this evidence, we do not need to keep the bones "completely" still.

There are many studies that are very clear at saying that some motion at the ends of the fractured bone may in fact help in healing. Apparently, in the early stages of healing (first 4-6 weeks), mechanically moving the ends of the fracture in an axial direction (IE separating the fracture apart and letting it come back together) just a small distance (.2 mm to 2 mm) is actually beneficial to, and speeds up, bone repair.

Moving the bone larger distances apart seems to slow down healing, as does moving the bones using shear (side to side movement), torsion (twisting) or bending the bone.

The research that focuses on the motion between the ends of the fractured bone segments (Inter Fragmentary Motion - IFM) is very difficult to do, because every fracture has a whole list of factors that are unique to that specific injury, making comparisons difficult.

In fact, from one study in Norway (done with rabbits), it is clear that slight motion at the fracture site is one of the primary factors in rapid healing (and in the strength of the healed bone). The researchers broke (then repaired with an internal plate) the tibia of a whole batch of (19) rabbits. Ten were left to heal with only the plate (group A), the other rabbits also received a cast immobilizing their leg (group B). After 6 weeks, all of the rabbits were killed and their tibias were dissected to see how well the breaks had healed (compared to the normal tibias). Interestingly, those rabbits without the cast (group A) had bones, which were at 107% of normal strength. Those rabbits in group B (with the cast) had tibia that were at 55% of normal strength. The researchers concluded that the most likely cause of delayed healing was the reduced function of the muscles, which led to a decreased blood flow to the fracture area.

NASA has found that astronauts will develop atrophy of their muscles in as little as 3 days without gravity (and therefore strain on the muscle system), if they are not doing exercises to prevent the atrophy. So, we are talking about a very quick degeneration of the muscles (and the bone), if there is complete immobilization.

In other studies (also done with rabbits with non-fractured bones), joint immobilization caused radical muscle atrophy and bone loss. The lack of muscular action is thought to be the most important factor in causing bone atrophy. There was a reduction in femoral bone strength by one third after immobilization of the hind limb (of the rabbits) in a plaster cast for 6 weeks.

It is interesting to note that the actual strength of the bone is significantly affected by the use of the muscles around that bone.

From these studies we can conclude that complete immobilization should be avoided, as it may in fact slow down the healing of the fracture. One can see why for a simple fracture a basic cast (which does not provide perfect immobilization) can promote healing better than complete immobilization (which would require a longer time of physical therapy to repair the atrophy degeneration caused by immobilized muscles, as well as the reduced blood flow to the area caused by non-used muscles).

With this research in mind, we can see that we do not need to "baby" the repairing limb with complete immobilization. Minor motion is not only acceptable, but beneficial, not only for the actual fracture repair itself, but also with the repair/health of the surrounding muscles and soft tissue. If the surrounding muscles can be used (at least minimally) during the early and mid-stages of the bone repair, the amount of time needed for repair of the complete injured system (bone, cartilage, muscle, tendons, ligaments, etc.) is reduced.

Ultimately, what allows the body to heal the fracture of the bone is the flow of blood to that injured area. The better the blood flow to the injured area, the quicker the injury will be healed.

The analogy to think of is a construction site in a busy city. When a construction project is undertaken, there are an enormous amount of materials that first need to be removed (dirt, ruble, old buildings, damaged cells, damaged bone, etc.). This normally occurs using bulldozers and back-hoes, which put all of the material to be removed into large dump trucks. These dump trucks need an exit path to take the rubble, trash and by-products of construction to a dump site far removed from the construction site. The waste needs to be removed or construction will grind to a standstill.

At the same time, all of the new raw materials need to be brought in to the construction site. Cement trucks will be coming in with raw cement. Large trucks will be arriving with steel and wood and other raw building materials. There is a constant influx of materials in order for any construction to occur.

Your blood flow is the transportation highway to and from the "re-construction" site (bone fracture). If the blood flow is constricted or reduced in any way, the repair will take longer (or not occur at all). If blood flow to an injured area is shut off completely, that injured area will simply die.

After the fracture and initial blood clot forms, tiny blood vessels begin to immediately work their way into that blood clot in order to provide blood flow. Anything that keeps the blood flow from beginning or continuing well is destructive and counterproductive to a rapid repair of the fracture. Many of the lifestyle issues that we will be discussing are counterproductive to a quick fracture repair, because they decrease blood flow. Those things that increase blood flow, naturally speed up the repair of the bone. So, massages, exercise, hot tubs and whirlpools will generally be very good to increase blood flow and therefore to promote a quick recovery. This brings us to Protocol Two. Protocol Two should not be initiated, until the fracture has entered the Restorative Phase of bone healing (a fracture callus is already well developed) - possibly 3 to 4 days after the initial injury.

2. Protocol TWO: Increase the blood flow to the injured area

Principle: "Anything that increases the blood flow to the fracture site, without damaging the fracture callus, will promote and increase the speed of the bone repair." We will look at four primary methods of increasing the blood flow to the fracture site: Axial movement of the fracture, Physical Therapy, Massages/Whirlpools/Hydrotherapy, and micro motion Wave Therapy (Ultrasound/Electrotherapy).

A. Axial Movement IFM (Interfragmentary Movement)

We have already mentioned that the studies show that small micro-movements at the actual bone fracture site stimulate healing. The healing effect of this micro-movement is such an accepted principle that producers of bone splints now are making the splints with flexibility built in to the splints. There are flexible portions of the splints that are bolted to a damage bone. This flexibility allows slight movement of the fractured bone ends, and therefore increases the speed of fracture repair. Previously, these splints had been totally rigid, and had simply been bolted to the bones, not allowing any interfragmentary movement.

With these small improvements in hardware, bones now heal slightly faster.

For the purpose of this protocol, your procedure will be to somehow allow the bone ends to have enough interfragmentary movement, without damaging the callus. It is your "challenge" to figure out a way to move the bone ends apart slight distances (.2mm to 2mm) without bending them, twisting them, or allowing shear movement occur.

The controlled studies of bone movement tell us that if the fractured bone ends are bent more than 20 degrees on a consistent basis, then the callus itself will become larger and much more flexible. In other words, the repair will be much more like cartilage. It will actually create a larger, more flexible callus, but in the end, it will take longer to transform that callus into actual bone. Ultimate bone healing is not accelerated, even though the repair is very flexible sooner.

So, you will need to figure out a way that you can do minor micro-movements of the fractured bone ends. Most of the medical studies are using these micro-movements for 20 minutes a day or so. If someone is trying to replicate the results of these experiments on their own fracture site, they will need to keep in mind the limits of movement, and refrain from separating the fracture beyond the 2mm of movement - and of course, totally avoid the shear, twisting or bending of the fracture site.

One possible method someone could use to create micro-vibrations might be to use a personal vibrator or any vibrating type gizmo on the far end of the fractured bone. These vibrations should be less than 2mm, therefore limiting the movement at the fracture site to less than 2mm as well. An example of a vibrating machine would be a vibrating plate that one stands upon.

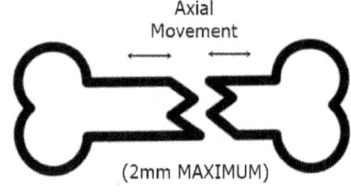

Any attempt at interfragmentary movement should be overseen by your healthcare provider, and of course, great care must be used, especially if there are multiple fractures or complications.

B. Physical Therapy

As soon as possible, after the fractured bone has been reduced and protected, physical therapy on the fractured bone site should begin. The sooner mobility is returned to the area, the sooner the body will heal the fracture. In fact, if there is ligament and tendon damage, as well as a fractured bone, there is a distinct possibility that the soft tissue repair may take longer than the actual bone repair.

Some serious fractures may need to hold off on physical therapy, but in general, the sooner that you can work to return mobility to the joints around the fracture, the quicker the complete injury will heal.

When we are talking about physical therapy, we are talking about moving the muscles and joints on both sides of the fracture site, but not directly on the fracture site itself. For instance, if a forearm bone has been broken (radius or the ulna), then the physical therapy would initially concentrate on the movement at the hand and the shoulder. When the pain level has decreased, then the physical therapy should begin with the wrist joint and the elbow joint. Joints should not be immobilized long term, if at all possible. Remember the damage that can happen from complete immobility in as little as three days. The immobility CAUSES this damage. You must return to using your joints and muscles as quickly as possible.

Weight-bearing physical therapy exercises should not begin, until you have been cleared for them, thru your healthcare physician. Normally, the physician will initially classify the injury as non-weight bearing (NWB). Then, the healthcare provider may allow you partial weight bearing (PWB), and then on to weight bearing as tolerated (WBAT), and finally they will allow full weight bearing (FWB). The goal is to begin moving weight on to the damaged limb, as quickly as possible (while still protecting it from further damage). Once you have been cleared to apply weight bearing as tolerated (WBAT), you are to use your pain as a guide, as to how much weight to put on the healing bone. Remember, the goal is to NOT re-damage the callus. You should begin putting weight on the bone, but at the same time, you should be very careful to not re-injure the broken bone.

It is true that high impact stress on the bones (from running or jumping) does indeed increase the bone density, and strengthen our bones. In the case of an injury being repaired, however, we do NOT want to use high impact "jarring" of the bone during the healing process. The likelihood of damaging the callus, and causing a delay in healing is too great. These "high impact" exercises should be avoided in the healing phase of the fracture. They should, however, be implemented in any strategy of long term bone strength/health. We will look at a strategy for long term bone health later in this report.

Muscle exercise of the surrounding joints of a fracture will increase the blood flow to the area (which increases the speed of healing). Any muscular exercises distal (beyond the fracture site) should be exercised soon after the fracture has been professionally stabilized, and often, if these exercises do not cause pain to the fracture. You would not want to begin exercises while the initial blood clot is still forming at the fracture site, but within a few days of the injury, the callus should be ready to get heavy blood flow.

For example, if the humerus is fractured (the upper arm bone), then exercises of the hand and wrist would be able to begin, as soon as your pain threshold will allow it. The exercising of the hand and wrist put no strain at all on the stability of the humerus, and those distal exercises will significantly increase the amount of blood flowing to the fracture site (and beyond….to feed the muscles in the hand and wrist).

Another benefit of rigorous exercise during fracture recovery is that exercise not only increases blood flow throughout the whole body, but it also signals our body to produce HGH (human growth hormone). This HGH occurs naturally whenever we exercise, and will be carried to all parts of the body. Of course, this natural HGH will stimulate growth at the fracture site (where it is needed). So, exercise of the whole body or other parts of the body from the fracture have a beneficial effect on rapidly healing the fracture.

Nothing stated above should be construed, so that anyone should think it is acceptable to "play through" a broken bone injury. NEVER continue to use a broken bone. If the bone is not protected and allowed to heal, the continual re-damaging of the fracture callus will increase the amount of time needed to heal the bone. If a broken bone is not protected and allowed to heal, it is possible for the bone to NEVER heal…. To become what is known as a "non-union." Do not think that you can tough it out, and play "just a few more times." NO…. When the fracture occurs, you MUST STOP using the injured bone immediately…. And start at the beginning with the complete "Rapid Bone Repair Protocol."

C. Massages/Whirlpool/Contrast Hydrotherapy

The recurring principle is that anything that protects the healing bone from damage (through shear, bending, twisting or LARGE axial movements), and yet increases the blood flow, will accelerate healing. Beyond range of motion and actual exercises that are done with physical therapy, there are other methods of increasing the blood flow to the damaged area.

Massages are a legitimate way to increase the blood flow to a specific area of the body. Massaging the areas distal to the fracture will certainly increase blood flow to and past the fracture site, and therefore accelerating healing. Massaging on the fracture site itself must be done with extreme care, and will initially be quite painful, but after the callus has formed, there would not be much danger of damaging the callus, if care was used in the massing of the fracture site itself. At this time, massaging the callus itself has not been studied in clinical trials, but the general principles clearly apply. If the bone is protected from further damage, AND the blood flow is increased at the fracture site, the healing will be accelerated.

The whirlpool is basically massaging something, using hot or warm water under pressure. After the initial callus is formed (3 or 4 days), using a whirlpool to gently massage beyond (distal to) the fracture site is a legitimate treatment option. Of course, the same rules apply. Care must be taken to not do any further damage to the healing callus by causing any shear, twisting, bending or large axial movements.

When pain tolerance will allow, gentle whirlpool therapy can begin at the actual fracture site.

To this date, there are no known controlled clinical studies showing that whirlpool therapy helps increase the speed of fracture healing, but there are many that show whirlpool treatment does indeed help decrease swelling, and also helps in the reduction of pain. This type of therapy will certainly increase the blood flow to the site stimulated, and so should certainly be used, even in the absence of definitive clinical "proof."

Contrast hydrotherapy is a method of alternating cold and hot water on an affected limb (or actually the whole body). It has been used for many years as a treatment for all types of injuries, and for general health immunity. There have been many clinical trials on contrast hydrotherapy, and the evidence supports the fact that alternating hot and cold water on an injury site certainly does something, though the results of the studies do not decisively prove anything definitively. The evidence does seem to show that contrast hydrotherapy can decrease recovery time after physical exercise, but no real studies have looked at how it affects a healing fracture.

Because there are no authoritative studies (yet) does not mean that we cannot use the therapy. It certainly does seem that alternating hot and cold water on an affected limb would indeed increase the blood flow to the limb. This increased blood flow is what we want to stimulate. Alternating hot and cold water could easily be done carefully without putting any damaging forces on a fracture callus. Shear, twisting, bending and large axial movements could be avoided during these hot/cold water treatments.

It is also possible to increase the blood flow to a fracture site by doing hydrotherapy to the opposite limb. For instance, if the right ankle is broken, and for some reason cannot be immersed in alternating hot/cold water….then the opposite ankle can be treated. Blood flow, even in this instance, increases to the damaged ankle.

D. Wave Therapy (Ultrasound and Electrotherapy)

Both ultrasound and electromagnetic therapy would cause micro-vibrations and micro-movements of the bone ends and the callus. It would follow from our general principle that they should contribute in helping a bone to heal.

(LIPUS) Low Intensity Pulsed Ultrasound is an FDA approved method (in 1994) of treating soft tissue and skeletal injuries. It is increasing in popularity, and will become much more popular in the medical field, as practitioners acquire the machines, and become more comfortable prescribing them for use in injury repair. Side effects are minimal to non-existent.

Ultrasound has been used and studied for years in the treatment of "non-unions" (a fractured bone that has refused to re-connect). Recently, they have begun to be studied and used with "regular" fractures, and do indeed show promise as a regular and effective treatment, which will help in the repair process of a fractured bone. There have been 7 definitive studies on LIPUS and bone repair. Three of those studies showed significant benefit and speed in fracture repair, while 4 of the studies do not show any increase. One of the factors that might explain why the 4 studies do not show any increase in rehabilitation time is that those studies didn't start the ultrasound until after the 4th week. It might be that the ultrasound has its most dramatic effects when started early and continued through the whole healing process.

In fact, three of the studies had a dramatic difference in length to rehabilitation. Using the LIPUS procedure, the length to recovery averaged 11 weeks, but those who received the placebo treatment had recoveries averaging 20 weeks. This is a dramatic difference in time between the two groups, and the medical researchers are optimistic that LIPUS is a beneficial procedure, which needs more controlled studies.

In the meantime, before the authoritative data is all in, due to the free market, there are new portable LIPUS machines that are available online for $60 to $100 dollars. All of the studies used the same parameters, so if you are going to be using LIPUS, use these parameters: a 30-mW/cm2 intensity, 1.5-MHz frequency repeated at 1 kHz, and a pulse width of 200 μs administered for 20 minutes each day.

The exact mechanism of how and why the ultrasound is beneficial is still not fully known, but many believe that the benefits are mechanical in nature. In other words, the micro-vibrations at the molecular level instigate the healing processes, and therefore, speed up bone healing. In any case, it is a safe procedure that MAY be very helpful in the healing process.

Electrotherapy is also used to speed up bone healing. It is a machine that sends small electrical charges into the muscles (or bone), stimulating contraction in the muscles, and potentially stimulating bone healing at a fracture site. Again, this procedure is accepted by the FDA and many clinics, and physical therapy offices will have and use these devices.

Studies have been going on for over 60 years, and, in general, the findings are encouraging. One author (D. Paterson) is as bold as to state: *"It has been proved that electrical stimulation produces osteogenesis (bone regeneration). Orthopedic surgeons should no longer be skeptical about this."*

In fact insurance companies now offer Electrotherapy in cases of bone non-union, and in certain other "difficult" fracture cases. They acknowledge that electrotherapy has a healing effect, but since most fractures eventually heal without the electrical stimulation, why include it for every treatment? Therefore, the therapy is only available for difficult fracture cases or "non-unions."

So here we have another therapy that helps in fracture repair, but is not covered by most insurance companies (for budgetary reasons). This only makes sense. The insurance company is concerned with your fracture repair, but NOT generally concerned with your RAPID bone repair.

Fortunately, there are machines available to the knowledgeable consumer that will allow treatment at home. In fact, some of these machines are combo machines that include both electrotherapy and ultrasound in the same portable machine. These dual purpose machines are available online for under $130. They are sometimes marketed as "muscle stimulators."

The original principle that is the basis of protocol 2 remains: "Everything that increases the blood flow to the fracture site, without damaging the fracture callus, will promote and increase the speed of the bone repair." Many of these other procedures may do much MORE than increase the blood-flow, but they at LEAST increase the blood-flow, and should, therefore, be thoughtfully considered by you and your healthcare provider, for inclusion in your own personal treatment plan.

3. Protocol THREE: Sleep 8 to 10 hours each night

Your body is in overdrive, working "like a dog" to repair the fractured bone. It makes sense that sleep is absolutely necessary as a stimulating factor in rapid bone repair.

There have been multiple studies on sleep and wound healing, but they show mixed results. Some studies show sleep patterns positively affect the time it takes for a wound to heal, other show no improvement at all.

One study on rats in Wisconsin did show that long term sleep deprivation caused significant damage to the bone health of rats in the study. Bone strength was affected, osteoblast count were decreased, among other findings. The authors concluded: *"these findings suggest that chronically inadequate sleep affects bone metabolism and bone marrow composition, in ways that have implications for development, aging, bone healing and repair, and blood cell differentiation."*

Sleep is also one of the few known times when your body produces and releases HGH (human growth hormone), which is definitely a factor in increasing the rate of your fracture repair. Any natural HGH that your body produces will be directed to the area of need (your fracture site).

Sleep may also be a mitigating factor on Stress levels. Of course, stress levels will be elevated when and if you have a fractured bone, but studies have shown that high levels of stress significantly slow down healing. Regular and sufficient sleep after a fracture will ensure that the stress levels are at least minimized, so as not to exacerbate (or lengthen) the bone healing process.

This step in the protocol is the easiest one to perform. You can start tonight and continue until the fracture is completely healed.

These three physical protocols are the cornerstone of quick fracture repair. Protecting the fracture site, increasing the blood flow to the fracture site, and getting enough sleep are all essential in the healing process. Next, we will look at the protocols that deal with things that we ingest, inhale or inject in one way or another, and how those "nutrients" or "chemicals" affect the rate of fracture repair.

B. Nutritional Recommendations

4.   Protocol FOUR: Immediately Stop These Four Things:

a. Smoking

Smoking has been shown to decrease blood flow. Enough said. The goal of this whole rapid bone repair protocol is to increase blood flow, which in turn will help the body to heal the fractured bone. Smoking decreases blood flow, thereby slowing down the healing process.

One meta-study looked at 974 clinical trials dealing with smoking and fractures. They compiled all of the data, and showed that smoking negatively affects bone healing. They point out that the overview "suggests smokers have a 40% increased time to union and 40% increased chance of non-union compared with non-smokers".

In another study of tibial fractures (the large upper leg bone), comparing time to complete healing, the researchers found that smokers took 269 days to heal, while non-smokers took 136 days to heal. That is almost twice as long, almost 100% more time.

I know these studies won't convince a committed smoker to give up smoking, but for those of you who need to rapidly heal a broken bone, these studies just might push you over the edge to a lifestyle change that you should really make.

b. Heavy Alcohol Use

Moderate alcohol use has been shown to have health benefits, but heavy alcohol usage negatively affects the body's ability to heal bones rapidly.

One study on rats with heavy alcohol use and fractured bones concluded that heavy alcohol use resulted in 26% less rigidity, 24% less intrinsic strength, and 14% less bone ash density of the repair tissue. These results are significant. Heavy alcohol use negatively affects fracture repair.

c. Heavy Sugar use

Heavy sugar use should be stopped immediately. Sugar is not one of those nutritious foods that will help your body in the healing process. In fact it does just the opposite.

Sugar has been shown to immediately and dramatically decrease the immune response system of your body. Researchers found that sugars reduce the phagocytic capacity of white blood cells (your immunity response). Phagocytic capacity is the ability of white blood cells to kill viruses, bacteria and remove foreign matter from the blood. In 1973, a scientific study, done by Albert Sanchez and colleagues at the Loma Linda University in California, found that oral ingestion of 100 gm of sugar (2 sodas) from glucose, fructose, sucrose, honey, or orange juice significantly reduced the capacity of neutrophils to engulf bacteria. They found that the greatest suppression happened between 1 to 2 hours after consumption, and was significant even 5 hours after feeding. The same study found that ingesting the same amount of starch (complex carbohydrates, which your body turns into glucose) did not affect the immune system in the same way.

Sugar is clinically linked to diabetes, heart disease, premature aging, what is now known as "metabolic syndrome," weakened immune system, and many other chronic and short term illnesses. There have been over 8000 medical and scholarly studies, and the results are not mixed. They consistently agree by showing damage being caused to the human body after ingesting sugar. The only real debate is "how much is too much?" In other words, everyone agrees that refined sugar is an insult to the human body, but everyone is trying to figure out how to have as much of it as possible.

One 12 can or bottle of soda contains more sugar than any adult should ingest in one day. Period. That doesn't include all of the added-in extra sugar from condiments, dressings, soups, prepared foods, etc.

Suffice it to say. When you are trying to help your body repair a traumatic "fracture", you should cut out any "extra" sugar at all.

Extra sugar can be considered anything that is significantly designed around sweeteners, such as sodas, desserts, sports drinks, candies, chocolates, fruit juices, honey, ice cream, etc. They ALL slow down the healing process. Sugar that is found in bread, mayonnaise, ketchup, mustard, some (non-sweet) dressings, soups, etc. are almost impossible to track down and eliminate from a diet, so allow them to remain. No need to go "crazy" and become a "sugar-phobic" or a "sugar-nazi", but at the same time, ANY foods designed specifically around sugar should be immediately eliminated from your diet, until the fracture has been completely healed.

Of course it would be best to continue eliminating those "extra" sugar foods from your diet completely. Your health will absolutely be improved. Actually, if this single change were made in the standard "American" diet, dramatic health improvement would immediately follow across the board.

d. Aspirin, Ibuprofen, or "Aleve"

In the past few years, there have been multiple medical studies that show that Non-Steroidal Anti-Inflammatory Drugs (NSAID's) delay fracture repair. They should be avoided initially AND throughout the complete duration of the fracture repair.

The authors summarize their findings, *"In summary, non-steroidal anti-inflammatory drugs inhibit osteoblasts in the early phases of bone-healing. These drugs exert an inhibitory action on fracture repair in animal models. They have been found to cause a delay in fracture-healing. It may be prudent for patients to avoid non-steroidal anti-inflammatory drugs following osseous (bone) injury"*.

An NSAID's list to avoid include the following drugs:

Aspirin (Anacin, Ascriptin, Bayer, Bufferin, Ecotrin, Excedrin)
Choline and magnesium salicylates (CMT, Tricosal, Trilisate)
Choline salicylate (Arthropan)
Celecoxib (Celebrex)
Diclofenac potassium (Cataflam)
Diclofenac sodium (Voltaren, Voltaren XR)
Diclofenac sodium with misoprostol (Arthrotec)
Diflunisal (Dolobid)
Etodolac (Lodine, Lodine XL)
Fenoprofen calcium (Nalfon)
Flurbiprofen (Ansaid)
Ibuprofen (Advil, Motrin, Motrin IB, Nuprin)
Indomethacin (Indocin, Indocin SR)
Ketoprofen (Actron, Orudis, Orudis KT, Oruvail)
Magnesium salicylate (Arthritab, Bayer Select, Doan's Pills, Magan, Mobidin, Mobogesic)
Meclofenamate sodium (Meclomen)
Mefenamic acid (Ponstel)
Meloxicam (Mobic)
Nabumetone (Relafen)
Naproxen (Naprosyn, Naprelan*)
Naproxen sodium (Aleve, Anaprox)
Oxaprozin (Daypro)
Piroxicam (Feldene)
Rofecoxib (Vioxx)
Salsalate (Amigesic, Anaflex 750, Disalcid, Marthritic, Mono-Gesic, Salflex, Salsitab)
Sodium salicylate (various generics)
Sulindac (Clinoril)
Tolmetin sodium (Tolectin)
Valdecoxib (Bextra)

Notice that the list to avoid does NOT include acetaminophen (Paracetamol; Tylenol). Acetaminophen relieves pain by elevating the pain threshold, that is, by requiring a greater amount of pain to develop, before it is felt by a person. It can safely be taken in all stages of your fracture repair, without inhibiting the repair process.

Now that we have looked at some of the chemicals and substances to AVOID during fracture repair, it is time to take a look at the nutrients and substances that we should INCREASE.

5. Protocol FIVE: Temporarily Increase Protein and Caloric intake (x3)

Your body is working overtime to repair a major trauma. Give it the calories and energy it needs to complete the process. You should immediately increase your caloric intake to three times (x3) your "normal" accepted caloric intake. If you normally eat 2500 calories, you should increase that to 7500 calories per day, until the fracture is significantly healed. This is a temporary elevation of calories for the purpose of insuring that the required proteins and "fuel" is available for your body to carry out the fracture repair. You should NOT be restricting calories, while your body is trying to repair a fractured bone.

Many studies show that low protein diets are correlated with weaker bones. When the protein levels in a diet are switched to a high protein diet, the strength and density of the bones also increases. In fact, one study concluded that, "dietary proteins are as essential as calcium and vitamin D for bone health."

Another study of elderly patients who had suffered hip fractures found that those with protein supplementation had an average hospital stay of 69 days, while those without the protein supplementation had an average hospital stay of 102 days. When all things are equal, other than protein intake and the protein group shows healing 35 days sooner… wow! How easy is that to fix!

Remember, this protocol is not a license to overeat or "gorge." It is a temporary increase of calories and protein, so that your body has the necessary materials and energy available to rapidly heal the fracture. When the fracture is completely healed, the caloric intake should return to the "normal" amounts (women: 1500-1900 calories and men: 2300-2500 calories). It would be wise to continue with a high protein diet for long term bone health (if there is the possibility of osteoporosis).

6. Protocol SIX: Temporarily "Shock-load" the Raw Structural Elements your body needs to repair the bone (x3)

We recommend three times the daily recommended amount of ALL of the structural elements that are required to build or "grow" bone. This includes all of the minerals found in bone, all of the proteins and amino acids found in cartilage, tendons and ligaments. Some of these raw structural elements are not even mentioned with a Daily recommended allowance, but the intake of those should be increased as well. From here on out, we will talk about an increase over the Daily recommended values of a mineral or a vitamin as a "Shock-load." We are recommending a Shock-load of essential minerals and other basic bone-building blocks.

We will be recommending a "Shock-load" of the vitamins, amino acids, proteins and other "co-factors" in the next protocol, but for now, we will stick with the essential structural elements that you   need to ingest.

These essential substances that any bone needs are Calcium,

Phosphorus, Magnesium, Collagen, Chitosan and Silica. These six substances can potentially be obtained from the diet, but to get them in the quantities that your body needs during the healing process would be difficult. It is much easier to get a good portion of these, using oral dietary supplements.

The body will need these elements in the basic percentages that occur in bones naturally. So, if you just started eating bones, you would go a long way towards fulfilling this protocol. And this makes sense, because your body is trying to "fill in the gap" between two fracture ends. Your body needs the specific minerals in the specific percentages that are found in bone and cartilage. This principle seems almost self-intuitive, yet is currently far from the accepted "knowledge." As a matter of fact, there are still medical practitioners, for whatever reason, that may even say that supplemental minerals and vitamins are a "waste of time and money." DO NOT LISTEN TO THEM. In fact, the medical studies of the past 50 years have been consistently showing how beneficial these minerals and vitamins are to health in general, and bone health in particular.

A natural and popular method of getting these nutrients that folks have recently begun talking about is eating what is known as "bone broth." This bone broth is a great idea and highly recommended. It can be inexpensively made at home, or purchased pre-prepared. Basically, "bone broth" is simply beef, poultry or fish bones that have been boiled and simmered, until the minerals have come out into the "broth." You will have the minerals and amino acids in the correct proportion that your body needs them. Basically, the procedure for making bone broth is to get 2 pounds of good healthy bones, and then bring them to a boil. Once they are boiling, reduce the heat and simmer them for 8 hours (fish), 24 house (poultry) or 48 hours (beef). The resulting broth will be mineral and amino acid rich. If allowed to cool down to room temperature, it will solidify. This is not fat, it is collagen and the gelatinous amino acids that your body needs to repair any structural skeletal issue. This "broth" is NOT vegan or vegetarian, nor could it be. It would be best to consider temporarily becoming an "omnivore", if you are a vegan or vegetarian that is hoping for a "rapid bone repair." Of course, "chicken soup" has been used as a folk remedy for years. Maybe grandma knew what she was talking about!

These structural elements that your body needs to repair the bone are like the concrete blocks, the steel re-bar, and the poured concrete at a construction site. Make sure your body has plenty of them. Any excess supplies will not hurt the re-construction process, but lack of supplies will definitely slow down the repair process.

If your diet does not include enough of these raw structural building blocks, your body will leech these required elements from the other bones in your body. Your body is smart enough to know that the important place for these building blocks is at the fracture site, so it will remove calcium, phosphorus and other necessary "stuff" from other bones. This has been observed in multiple clinical studies and the test results show that other bones actually have a lower bone mineral density scan, and become "weaker." It is clear that your body will "rob from Peter to pay Paul." Of course, we do not want to weaken our other bones as the fracture heals; we want all of our bones to stay strong, or to get even stronger! To ensure this, we must supplement with these raw materials.

Shock-loading of raw minerals is a controversial idea, but one that makes sense in this case, for a temporary time period (until the bone fracture has completely healed). Also, we do not recommend any mineral "shock-loading" without also including protocol 7, which is to simultaneously "shock-load" the necessary co-factors that these elements need in order to be rendered "bio-available" by the body. In this limited circumstance, we wholeheartedly recommend elemental "shock-loading".

We will now look a little closer at the core essential elements that you should be shock-loading:

a. Calcium

Calcium makes up 66% of the mass of your bones. It is the primary structural mineral, and the medical establishment has grudgingly admitted that supplementing with Calcium is a good idea for long term bone health (they also grudgingly agree that Vitamin D and Vitamin K are beneficial "co-factors.") in females and males alike.

There are many forms of Calcium commercially available in supplemental form. Any Calcium is better than nothing, but there are some forms of Calcium that are more bio-available, and so come more highly recommended. We will be talking about these elements as "Good, Better, or Best."

Calcium is sold inexpensively as "Calcium Carbonate." This is commonly used as an "antacid". It is made by grinding up "limestone" or clamshells and looks like a chalky powder (or pill). It is not very bio-available, but your body can use it (assuming the necessary co-factors are present). It must be taken with food. Calcium Gluconate is simply calcium carbonate neutralized with gluconic acid. Also, not very bio-available. These forms of calcium are "better than nothing."

A better Calcium supplement that can be taken without food is Calcium Citrate.

A much more bio-available form of Calcium is "TriCalcium Phosphate". It is either derived from vertebrate bones or from certain rocks. Also known as "bone ash", this is used as a supplement or in surgical bone grafts (to actually mechanically fill in "voids" in bones that are vacant and need to be re-modeled). Recently, it has been used as a 3d printed scaffold that is surgically installed as a bone graft with promising results.

There are studies showing that Ossein Microcrystalline Hydroxyapatite (OHC) is a more effective form of supplemental Calcium than any of those mentioned above. This form of calcium can ONLY be produced from the bones of vertebrate animals. These bones are boiled down, filtered, purified, and therefore include not only calcium, but also all of the other minerals that are found in bone. Because of these extra minerals (as opposed to simply pure ground up "rock") the resulting supplement is very bio-available. This OHC is commonly used as a filler material for surgical bone graft (when a bone void needs to be filled), because it is so close to the physical make up of bone itself (as it is condensed bone itself). OHC is not vegan or vegetarian - it can't be. To get the nutrients of the bone requires animal bones from which to condense down the minerals. This is the BEST way to supplement calcium.

Do NOT think you can get the calcium that you need by drinking milk. In fact, one clinical study showed conclusively that milk does NOT help in bone health. In the experiment, mice were fed different diets before examining their skeletal health. The acidic casein (milk) supplemented mice exhibited poor mineral absorption and loose bone structure, whereas the neutralized casein or fermented milk supplemented mice were resistant to osteoporosis and had high bone mechanical properties. It seems clear that normal milk is not beneficial to bone health, and should not be counted on when increasing your calcium intake.

The amount of Calcium recommend as a daily intake by the FDA is 1000mg. Studies have shown that 50% of the population do NOT receive this recommended amount of calcium per day, from either diet or supplementation. Half of the population is under-nourished when it comes to calcium - by the FDA's own standards. And yet, many health care professionals for some reason will STILL not recommend a calcium supplement, even following a fracture!

During the shock-loading phase, we recommend at least 3000mg of the most bio-available calcium that you can acquire. You will not be able to get 3000mg of calcium from diet alone, so oral supplementation is required at this stage. Remember, you are also tripling the amount of calories that you are eating, so the increased caloric intake will also help in allowing your body to assimilate this shock-load of calcium.

You sometimes hear claims that your body can only use "natural" calcium from plants, but not calcium from "rocks." This is simply not true. Your body can break down and use any calcium, if it has the required co-factors that help with assimilation. Without these co-factors, ANY form of Calcium is not bio-available and potentially harmful. Any Calcium supplementation without the co-factors (explained in protocol 7) may actually be harmful to the body. Excess Calcium that is not bio-available can lead to health problems, including calcification of the arteries (which can be very serious).

b. Phosphorous

"Calcium without Phosphorous is Preposterous." The second leading mineral that makes up bone mass is Phosphorous. It works closely with Calcium, and the two are always "partners in crime." Any supplementation with Calcium should also include Phosphorous.

The normal daily allowance (700mg) of Phosphorous is typically obtained through the diet, but if in fact you will be Shock-loading Calcium, then you must also increase your intake of Phosphorous. The two minerals together are synergistic and the one cannot function without the other. The Merck Index states: "Phosphate is a major intracellular anion, which participates in providing energy for metabolism of substances, and contributes to important metabolic and enzymatic reactions in almost all organs and tissues. Phosphate exerts a modifying influence on calcium concentrations." The mineral is absolutely essential to the "rapid" healing process of a fracture, and should not be inadvertently overlooked. We recommend 800mg/day as a shock-load amount and 290mg/day for normal health maintenance.

c. Magnesium

Magnesium is important for many processes in the body, including regulating muscle and nerve function, blood sugar levels and blood pressure, and making protein, bone, and DNA. It has been shown to help decrease bone degeneration in those suffering from Osteoporosis, and if there is a deficiency of simply 50%, there are negative effects on bone health. This is one of the synergistic core elements that dramatically affect skeletal health.

The daily recommended allowance is 400mg, but research has shown that at least 15% of the population does not receive the daily recommended amount. Magnesium is important in over 300 chemical reactions in the body, and hundreds of enzymes require Magnesium ions in order to function. Because of its value to bone health it should be shock-loaded along with Calcium and Phosphorus. We recommend 1200mg/day as a shock-load, and 400mg/day for normal bone health maintenance.

d. Collagen

Collagen is simply the living flexible, fibrous cartilage that is part of the skeletal system. It is found inside your bones (giving them flexibility), as well as being the predominant material in the fracture callus that forms at every fracture site. It is the main constituent of skin, connective tissue, and the organic (living) substance of bones and teeth.

You can get your Collagen by eating cartilage, or by eating its refined cousin: Gelatin. Gelatin is a mixture of peptides and proteins produced by partial hydrolysis of collagen extracted from the skin, bones, and connective tissues of animals, such as domesticated cattle, chicken, pigs, horses and fish. It is a polypeptide containing three peptide chains, and rich in proline and hydroxyproline. Gelatin is used to firm up soups, or to make "jello." We do not recommend making and eating Jello, as most Jello packages are 50% sugar. We do recommend unflavored gelatin. You can purchase this at the supermarket and mix it in to a "supplemental shake." Again, apologies to the vegetarians, but this is by far the BEST way to get the Hydrolyzed Collagen your body desperately needs as it repairs the fracture.

One meta-study concludes: "preclinical studies show that HC (Hydrolyzed Collagen) stimulates collagenic tissue regeneration by increasing not only collagen synthesis, but minor components (glycosaminoglycans and hyaluronic acid) synthesis as well. Clinical studies show that HC continual ingestion helps to reduce and prevent joint pain, bone density loss and skin aging. These results, as well as its high level of tolerance and safety, make HC ingestion attractive for a long-term use in bone and joint degenerative diseases and in fight against skin aging."

A side benefit of consuming this Collagen will be the increase in finger nail strength and growth, a decrease in joint pain, the increase in hair strength and growth, and the decrease of any wrinkles that you have on your skin. Not a bad list of side effects.

Of course, the best bone supplements will include Collagen or Gelatin in their ingredient list, as these raw materials are so vitally important to skeletal health.

We recommend at least 2400mg/day as a shock-load, and 800mg/day for regular bone health maintenance.

e. Chitosan

Chitosan or Chitin is an amide that forms the outer coverings of insects and crustaceans (shrimp, lobster). It is used in the structure of cell walls, and has been clinically shown to be very important in the process of bone re-generation. In the past 10 years, the medical community has started researching and using it in wound healing and bone regeneration. The results have been very positive. In fact, one study concludes that chitosan powder used as a "bone graft" material, "can be used to promote bone repair in situations where rapid bone regeneration is of high importance.".... Like YOURS!

In another study, Chitosan and Phosphorus together "increased vascularization of the provisional repair tissue, and increased intramembranous bone formation and subchondral bone remodeling." In other words, it improved the blood flow to the injury, AND it improved the bone healing process.

There is no official recommended daily amount of Chitosan, but we recommend at least 300mg daily in the "shock-loading" required for a rapid fracture repair. For normal bone maintenance, the daily amount should be reduced back to 100mg per day.

f. Silica

Silica (Silicon) has been shown to have an effect on bone calcification and mineralization. This element has been previously thought to have only negative health effects, but is now being studied for its positive impact on bone health.

In fact, two studies have reported the relationship between dietary silicon intake and osteoporosis. In both studies, increased silicon intake correlated with increased bone mineral density for men, premenopausal women, and post-menopausal women.

Again, with Silicon there is no official daily recommended intake amount, but we recommend at least 6mg of Silica in the shock-loading stage.

Many of these elements (and the vitamins we will be covering in the next section) are synergistic and work with each other. This is the reason that official clinical studies can neither confirm nor deny the benefits of many of these individual elements and vitamins. Is it prudent to wait around until there have been clinical studies that authoritatively prove the benefits of each individual mineral and vitamin before we use them? Absolutely not. Many of these minerals and vitamins are known to be beneficial in synergy with other minerals and vitamins. For us, to put our health on hold and wait until medical studies clinically "prove" these synergies before we use the supplements would be ridiculous. We can, and should, use common sense, as we approach our health, and try to help our bodies along by using an "all of the above" philosophy, because we know that many of these minerals and vitamins work synergistically.

Calcium, Phosphorus, Magnesium, Collagen, Chitosan and Silica are all important to the structural health of the skeletal system. There are many vitamins and minor minerals that are co-factors in making these structural elements much more bio-available. We will look at these co-factors in the next protocol.

7. Protocol SEVEN: Temporarily "Shock-load" the Necessary Co-Factors

These "Co-Factors" should never be left out when taking the primary structural elements that we talked about in protocol six. Any supplementation of Calcium, Phosphorus and Magnesium without these Co-Factors can in fact be dangerous to the health. Never shock-load elemental minerals without also shock-loading these important nutritional Co-Factors.

These Co-Factors are listed in general order of importance. This does not mean that the Zinc, Vanadium and Vitamin C can be skipped. Someone has to be last. No, these nutrients are still important, and should not be ignored, it's just that there is much more clinical evidence and clinical support for the Vitamins and Minerals, which are covered here first. In fact, Vitamin D3 and Vitamin K2 should ALWAYS accompany any calcium consumed.

a. Vitamin D3

Vitamin D is vitally important for calcium and phosphorus homeostasis and musculo-skeletal health. In children, severe vitamin D deficiency manifests as rickets, and vitamin D inadequacy can impair or retard attainment of peak bone mass. In adults, inadequate vitamin D can result in secondary hyper-parathyroidism, decreased Bone Mass Density, osteoporosis (fragility of bones - more "porous"), osteomalacia (softening of bones), and increased risk of fragility fractures. The medical community has "grudgingly" admitted that the studies do in fact conclude that Vitamin D is a required co-factor in conjunction with calcium to stimulate bone health. Multiple studies and clinical trials have shown that an inadequate Vitamin D level is probably the best indicator of poor bone health.

Hundreds of clinical trials (most including Calcium) have shown a correlation of Vitamin D (and Calcium) with skeletal health. There are some conflicting studies, but the vast majority of them point to Vitamin D deficiency as being an epidemic, and directly having negative health effects.

Fortunately, Vitamin D can be received by exposure of the bare skin to sunlight. Many folks who are bed-ridden or cannot get out in the sun for some reason or another (IE wintertime blues) are significantly deficient in Vitamin D. So, they need to supplement Vitamin D.

We recommend at least 800IU of Vitamin D3 per day supplemented. One can get much more Vitamin D from exposure to the sun, but that "sun supplied Vitamin D" is all a bonus, you should be getting at least 800IU of D3 supplementation for normal health (including bone health). In 2006 in the American Journal of Clinical Nutrition, Houghton and Vieth argue convincingly that the Vitamin D3 (cholecalciferol) is much more bio-available, efficacious and beneficial to health than the more common Vitamin D2 (ergocalciferol). Clinically, the tests show that D3 is at least three times more potent that D2, and that it stays in the body for up to 3 times longer! In fact, looking at all of the available clinical evidence, they conclude that Vitamin D2 should NOT even be regarded as a suitable supplement AT ALL! Their argument is persuasive, but to this day Vitamin D2 is still the most prescribed type of Vitamin for Osteoporosis or bone health. We recommend ONLY Vitamin D3. Do not supplement with the low quality & common Vitamin D2.

b. Vitamin K2

Vitamin K2 has been studied for the past 45 years and the evidence reveals that it is essential for keeping calcium IN bones and teeth, while keeping the calcium OUT of the arteries and soft tissues. This is a major issue, because calcium in the arteries (calcification) is a danger that is associated with calcium (obviously). So… when we recommend shock-loading calcium, we MUST include Vitamin K2, which helps keep the calcium in the skeletal system and out of the arteries. Without also supplementing Vitamin K2, we do NOT recommend shock-loading calcium.

In a clinical study in 2015 over in Japan, Inaba, Sato and Yamashita did a randomized, double blind study on Vitamin K and bone health. They found that daily Vitamin K intake improved bone metabolism, increased bone mineral density and bone strength, while decreasing fracture risk. They also found that Vitamin K is a co-factor in processing at least 14 K-dependent Gla-proteins. These proteins include osteocalcin, a bone modulator that binds to hydroxyapatite and helps it bind to bone, and Gla-protein, which inhibits vascular calcification. The results of their study resulted in the increase in the "official" recommended daily amount of K2 (for Japanese adults) to 100mg/day for normal bone health or 250-300mg/day for the prevention or treatment of osteoporosis. (NOTICE: how the official recommendations are in two stages, a "normal amount" for maintenance AND a "shock-load" amount for treatment of Osteoporosis. Just pointing out how that mirrors this current "Rapid Bone Repair Protocol" recommendations.)

There are two types of K2 Vitamins: menaquinone-4 (MK4) and menaquinone-7 (MK7). In 2012, researchers did a clinical study comparing the two types of Vitamin K. They discovered that MK7 is much more bio-available than MK4 and should be used exclusively. We recommend MK7 as the Vitamin K2 that is supplemented, and not the less effective (and cheaper) MK4.

Vitamin K2 is not normally accessible from the diet (unless your diet is very high in kale, collards or spinach). The only way to get this Vitamin in the required dosages is to supplement, even more so as you attempt to shock-load.

c. Fulvic Acid

Fulvic Acid is a type of Humic Acid that is formed from decaying vegetation. The most potent forms are found by mining the compressed leftover debris from ancient vegetation. This vegetation (from ages past) was mineral rich, and the resulting deposits contain multiple amino acids, over 70 trace minerals, and other organic acids. We know that organic fulvic acids are created by micro-organisms in the soil, for the purpose of transporting minerals and nutrients from the soil into the plant. Fulvic Acid chelates and prepares the raw elements to be accepted and used by our body's cells.

These mined fulvic acids have been used throughout recorded history for their medicinal properties with impressive results. In fact, in the Himalayan Mountains a substance known as Shulijat (Shilajit, mumie, vegetable asphalt, mineral pitch), which consists of over 40% Fulvic Acid, has been used as a treatment for genitourinary (old age) diseases, diabetes, digestive disorders, high altitude remedy, nervous diseases, tuberculosis, chronic bronchitis, asthma, anemia, eczema, bone fractures, and other diseases. It is known as a stimulator of bone regeneration in both the Russian and the Indian systems of health and medicine. It is now being studied in "the West" so that potential drugs can be produced (and sold) from the natural substance.

We all have heard of people living high in the mountains, eating only "yak yogurt" that live well past 100 years of age... Fulvic acids are thought to be one of the active ingredients in that lifestyle.

These Fulvic Acids have been studied for past 40 years or so, and the results of some of the studies are intriguing to say the least. In one experiment, patients who required the replacement or transplantation of bone were treated using fulvic acid as part of the therapy. Animal bone in the form of calcium hydroxyapatite, an inorganic calcium compound, was used in the "transplant." Normally neither animal bones nor inorganic calcium are readily absorbed by the human body. However, when fulvic acid was physically inserted into the animal bone before replacement, the patients experienced dramatically improved regeneration of the transplanted bones. The fulvic acid was so readily accepted and used by the patients that their bodies became highly osteoconductive. This means that new bone tissue began to form at an accelerated pace, thereby enhancing growth and healing. The inorganic calcium was also absorbed by the body, due to the fact that the fulvic acid had transformed it into an organic compound. At the end of the experiment, it was noted that in those control transplants without the introduction of fulvic acid into the bone tissues, healing was NOT accelerated and regeneration did not take place at the same pace.

Because Fulvic Acids chelate (make a compound by physically binding with) minerals, so that it transforms them into a bio-available form that our body can use, it can be used as a very potent co-factor in delivering these bio-available minerals, so that your body can readily repair the broken bone. These results are handed down through folk remedies, and they are now being demonstrated through clinical trials.

In November 2002, in the publication "Drug Development Research", Kwon and his fellow researchers explain how Fulvic Acid combined with human cells dramatically increases the osteoconductivity of the bone cells. They conclude that *"the data suggest that mumie is a potent stimulator of osteoblastic differentiation of mesenchymal stem cells and inhibitor of osteoclastogenesis, hence it may be of clinical benefit in the treatment for osteoporosis in humans."* In other words, it helps bones heal quickly and efficiently. These early studies have not resulted in a "marketable" drug for bone healing YET, but you and I can benefit from using Fulvic Acid BEFORE it has been turned into an official "drug."

In the past 15 years, study after study has been regularly released, each one talking about how Fulvic acid (in one of its forms) actually is beneficial for the treatment of_____ "blank"___.   These clinical studies include those benefits already listed, but also include many others, such as cognitive disorders - memory help (IE potential Alzheimer's treatment), helping with ulcers, having powerful antiviral benefits (against herpes, 1 & 2, HCMV, RSV, and VSV), it helps the immune system (has immunomodulatory effects), has an anti-allergy effect, has an anti-aging effect, has anti-inflammatory effects, helps with oxidative stress (is an anti-oxidant), is anti-radical, increases fertility (in rats), and is beneficial in treating "long term" wounds.

Many drugs have already reached the market that have been developed out of "Humic Acid." These include, but are not limited to: Shilagen, Abana, Cystone, Diabecon 400, EveCare, Geriforte, Lukol, Pilex, Rumalava, Tentex forte, Nefrotec, Adrenotone, Siotone, La-Tone Gold, Andro-Surge, Solanova Libidoplex.

The knowledgeable observer can see that this "miracle drug" actually does have historical and medical backing as a rejuvenator. We include it in this protocol as a NECESSARY Co-factor and as the PRIMARY delivery system of the raw minerals, so that they are delivered "bio-available" and ready to be applied to the rapid healing taking place at the fracture site.

Fulvic Acid can be purchased online or at your local health food store. Make sure that you purchase from a reputable source and from a source where the Fulvic Acid is extracted using water (rather than using a chemical extraction process). Independent laboratory tests of the potency and concentration of the Fulvic Acid would also be helpful in determining where to get your Fulvic Acid from. Fulvic Acid is available as a liquid, a powder, or a pill.

d. Green Tea Powder

Another beneficial Co-Factor in bone health is Green Tea Powder. There have been many clinical studies which have noticed that those who drank Green or Black Tea had a higher BMD (bone mineral density) and less fractures. This interesting connection has led to a bunch of research on the interconnection between Green Tea and bone health.

A review article in 2013 concluded that, "The evidence from in vitro (test tube studies) and animal studies of various bone-loss models strongly suggests that tea polyphenols, especially GTPs (Green Tea Polyphenols), are effective in protecting against osteoporosis… Tea and its polyphenol components act by increasing bone mass, trabecular bone volume, number, and thickness and reducing trabecular separation, as well as by suppressing bone resorption and enhancing bone formation, resulting in greater bone strength."

The authors end by saying that "more study is needed," which is definitely true. But in the meantime, we recommend using Green Tea Extract as a supplement, because of its positive effect on bone health. We don't need a definitive clinical study before we can begin seeing the benefits from this nutrient in our immediate situation.

The polyphenols, a large group of plant chemicals that includes the catechins, are thought to be responsible for the health benefits that have traditionally been attributed to tea, especially green tea. A side benefit from supplementing with these polyphenols is that they are also being studied for their potential anti-cancer properties. The results are not conclusive, but ongoing studies reveal more benefits of these nutrients every year.

e. L-lysine

An amino acid that plays a major role in calcium absorption; building muscle protein; recovering from surgery or sports injuries, and in the body's production of hormones, enzymes, and antibodies.

In one study, published in the journal "Nutrition," Gennari and his co-authors took 15 healthy women and 15 women with osteoporosis and studied how supplementing with L-lysine affected the absorption rate of supplemental calcium. They found that, "L-lysine can both enhance intestinal Ca absorption and improve the renal conservation of the absorbed Ca. The combined effects may contribute to a positive Ca balance, thus suggesting a potential usefulness of L-lysine supplements for both preventive and therapeutic interventions in osteoporosis."

L-lysine is clearly a co-factor in helping calcium become bio-available to the body. We recommend shock-loading of 900mg/day during the "Rapid Bone Repair Protocol," and simple supplementation of 300mg/day during long term treatment for bone health (or Osteoporosis).

f. Vitamin B6

Vitamin B6 (Pyridoxine) has been shown through many studies to be an important co-factor in the formation of cartilage (which is what is needed at your fracture callus site).

In fact, a Vitamin B6 deficient diet fed to rats for 4 weeks shows a significant reduction in the crosslink formation of their skin and cartilage. Remember, the cartilage is what makes up 1/3 of the mass of the bone, and gives it the flexibility needed (to protect it from cracking like a dry twig). Without strong cartilage at the fracture callus, there will be a delay in healing at the fracture site.

There have been many studies with humans examining hip fracture rates and B6 intake levels. The results have been mixed. More precise studies need to be carried out. In the meantime (because you have no time to wait for those studies to be completed), we recommend supplemental shock-loading with 300mcg/day and bone maintenance supplementing of 100mcg/day.

g. Boron

A Trace mineral that should be included in any supplement program. There are a whole host of benefits that have been clinically attributed to Boron supplementation. In Fact, in 2015, Pizzorno did a review of the available medical literature, and includes these benefits of Boron supplementation: 1) strengthening of the bones, 2) increasing wound healing, 3) it improves the bodies use of estrogen, testosterone and Vitamin D, 4) it boosts magnesium absorption, 5) raises levels of antioxidant enzymes, 6) protects against pesticide-induced oxidative stress and heavy-metal toxicity, 7) improves the brains electrical activity, cognitive performance, and short-term memory for elders, 8) has demonstrated preventive and therapeutic effects in a number of cancers, such as prostate, cervical, and lung cancers, and multiple and non-Hodgkin's lymphoma, 9) may help ameliorate the adverse effects of traditional chemotherapeutic agents.

Clinical evidence of strengthening of the bones would be enough, but clearly this mineral has multiple benefits and should be included in any supplementation aimed at the skeletal system. We recommend shock-loading at 9mg/day and a long term bone maintenance supplemental level of 3mg/day.

h. Copper and Zinc

Copper and Zinc are trace elements that have been found to be beneficial to both cartilage formation and normal skeletal formation in humans and animals. Not much of each is needed, but there have been correlations found with each of these elements dietary deficiency and bone health.

One study in 2015 found that if copper ions were surgically

included in a chitosan scaffold implanted to "remodel" broken bones in rats, the results were 11 times greater than not having a scaffold, and twice as good as having simply a chitosan scaffold. For some reason, the copper at the fracture site doubled the bone tissue regeneration.

In 2010, Yamaguchi did a review of all of the medical studies dealing with Zinc and found that, "Zinc is an essential nutritional factor in the growth of humans and animals". He discovered that, "bone growth retardation is a common finding in various conditions associated with dietary zinc deficiency. Bone zinc content has been shown to decrease in aging, skeletal unloading, and postmenopausal conditions, suggesting its role in bone disorder. Zinc has been demonstrated to have a stimulatory effect on osteoblastic bone formation and mineralization; it stimulates cellular protein synthesis. The intake of dietary zinc causes an increase in bone mass. The oral administration of zinc has the restorative effect on bone loss under various pathophysiologic conditions including aging, skeletal unloading, calcium - and vitamin D - deficiency, arthritis, estrogen deficiency, diabetes, and fracture healing". His conclusion is that, "Zinc compounds may be designed as a new supplementation factor in the prevention and therapy of osteoporosis."

We recommend supplemental shock-loading of Copper at 9mg/day and Zinc at 30mg/day and supplemental maintenance of Copper at 3mg/day and Zinc at 10mg/day.

i. Manganese

Another important trace element that has been shown to benefit bone health. Studies with rats have found that Manganese supplementation increased the BMD (bone mineral density) and bone formation of the rats in the study (over non-supplemented rats). Also, in 2007, Chesnick and associates demonstrated that Manganese has a significant positive effect on calcium being taken up by the osteoblasts and deposited as bone.

Manganese is one of the trace element that must be ingested in balance. Without it, there are health issues (specifically bone issues), but too much Manganese can also be dangerous for the health. So balance is required with this mineral. Ingesting too much manganese from food is not really possible, as the cases of Manganese "toxicity" have come from breathing industrial waste vapors that include Manganese.

We do recommend orally supplementing Manganese in the "shock-loading" stage at no more than a "safe" 10mg/day. For normal daily bone health maintenance, we recommend 3mg/day.

j. Vanadium

Another trace element that is important (in small doses) for the skeletal system is Vanadium. Studies have shown its importance for bone reformation. In one study from 2012, Vanadium salt was injected at the actual fracture site of rats who had femoral fractures. Those with this Vanadium injection had a callus that had 200% more cartilage than the control group. At 4 weeks following the fracture, the Vanadium injected rats had bones that were 154% stronger than the control. So the Vanadium not only helped with the speed of repair of the fracture callus, but it also increased the ultimate strength of the fracture repair as well.

Again, as a trace element not much of this is required, but to NOT have it would be shortchanging your personal fracture repair. We recommend oral supplemental shock-loading with Vanadium at 40mcg/day and for general bone health maintenance 13mcg/day.

k. Vitamin C

Ascorbic Acid seems like a strange addition to the list of necessary co-factors for bone health, but it should absolutely be in the list. Vitamin C is needed for the growth and repair of tissues in all parts of your body; it is used by your body to: Form an important protein used to make skin, tendons, ligaments, and blood vessels, heal wounds and form scar tissue, repair and maintain cartilage, bones, and teeth, and to aid in the absorption of iron.

It has been medically established for years that the lack of vitamin C causes scurvy, a pathological condition leading to blood vessel fragility and connective tissue damage, due to failure in producing collagen, and, finally, to death as result of a general collapse. The connection of Vitamin C with collagen production and synthesis in the body is important for us with this specific protocol as we are concerned with increasing the production of collagen in the fracture callus and eventually inside the healed bone.

We recommend an oral supplementation shock-load of Vitamin C of 250mg/day, and an oral supplementation for bone health maintenance at 90mg/day.

Of course, ALL of these co-factors should be taken simultaneously, so that the benefits of each will work synergistically with the other necessary co-factors. There are other vitamins and minerals that affect bone health as well, but these are the CORE essential co-factors that should not be missed in your oral supplementation procedure.

I recommend a supplement in powder form as the most convenient way to "shock-load" the recommended nutrients. A powder is already finely ground, and therefore is fairly easy for the body to digest and assimilate. Liquid supplements are also highly bio-available, but the amount of calcium required for the shock-loading makes a liquid supplement problematic (the taste becomes a real issue). A powder supplement can quickly and easily be mixed into your favorite smoothie, yogurt or apple sauce, and can, therefore, be enjoyed without having to "gag it down" (Which is important if you are doing 3 smoothies a day during the shock-loading phase)

There are some good supplements out there, but for the highest quality bone health supplement available, we do recommend our official "Rapid Bone Repair™" supplement, which has every one of the nutrients mentioned in the exact required percentages that your body needs for optimal healing. You can find it on Amazon or at www.NaturalNutritionWorks.com. It is actually designed so that each daily serving is one scoop. So, a shock-load of the necessary nutrients would simply be 3 scoops per day. Those scoops could be all in one smoothie, or spread out over three smoothies during the day.

IV. Long Term Bone Health

Long term bone health can be achieved by dialing back the recommendations found in this "Rapid Bone Repair Protocol." The recommendations already given for healing a bone are the exact same for long term bone health. The only difference would be that you should NOT be shock-loading the supplements.

You should still be taking all of the necessary raw materials we have just listed that are necessary for bone health, and you should also be taking all of the co-factors that make those raw materials bio-available. This synthesis will keep your skeletal system in great shape, even into your advanced years.

One thing that needs to be modified when talking about long term bone health is that you should be mechanically loading your bones. In the protocol, we were very careful about not putting heavy loads on "healing" bones until they had been cleared for "load bearing" by your health care practitioner. For long term maintenance of healthy bones you must load the bones. I am not talking about static loads like swimming or biking, but about actual pounding and shocking of the bones through heavy weights, or jumping or running. Actually, striking the bones and loading them repeatedly has been shown to dramatically increase the strength of the bones.

We are not talking about jumping off the roof, but small, controlled jumps will do the trick. We need to use our bones (and our bodies) or we will lose them. "Use it or lose it." You have heard that saying before, and it is very relevant when dealing with bone and skeletal health (also muscular health). Bones are known to respond to the stimuli under which they are placed.

So, do not be afraid of "jarring" your bones. That "jarring" is what will make them stronger and keep them healthy. If you have not been physically active, you should begin a moderate exercise routine, which includes jogging, brisk walking or stair climbing. This habit will keep your bones strong, and also keep the bone mineral density (BMD) high. Furthermore, this exercise will help your muscular coordination, which in turn will protect you from falls.

Another exercise (or treatment) that can potentially keep up your bone mass and strength is called "whole body vibration (WBV)". It is an alternative to anaerobic exercise that we mentioned previously. In this whole body vibration, you would stand on a machine for a specific time period that vibrates and "shakes" you (and your bones). The thinking is that this "shaking" will, if not increase, at least maintain your bone mineral density and bone strength. Results of studies on this fairly new approach have been mixed, but generally show an increase in bone mineral density from consistent use.

Of course, any long term bone health exercise program should be reviewed and authorized by your health care physician.

V. Conclusion

Do not be discouraged by the seemingly long list of nutritional supplements that you should be taking to heal your broken bone. Many high quality supplements designed for bone health will have most of these nutrients included. Any lacking nutrients are normally available at the health food store or online.

Your rapid recovery is worth the financial investment of those supplements. You have already invested a large amount of time reading through the protocol. Now it is up to you to actually APPLY what you have learned. Knowledge is powerful and empowering! But, it won't do any good just sitting and thinking about it. You NEED to begin supplementing as quickly as possible to get your fracture repair into high gear!

Also, you need to keep your bone repair time frames realistic. You can legitimately double the speed of a fracture repair, but that is from what it would have taken, if you had not taken the action required in the "Rapid Bone Repair" protocol. In other words, from doing nothing. This protocol will beat "nothing" with a stick, and if you do BOTH the physical recommendations AND do the shock-loading of the supplements, you will be amazed at how fast you will heal. Any bone repair is certainly going to take some time, so stay realistic.... But, with the protocol you can realistically shave weeks, if not months, off the amount of time that a "normal" fracture repair would take.

And.... I would love to hear about your progress.... Your story! I know it will be inspiring for others who are also starting the process of "healing" a broken bone. You know how discouraging it is to be bedridden and immobile. How encouraging to be able to share your "rapid bone repair" story with those who are at the beginning of the whole process. Once you have healed you can share your story at www.RapidBoneRepair.com. I am looking forward to hearing it!

All the best!

Randy Velker

Appendix A

Randy's Story:

"I am NOT missing my Senior Year of Basketball!"

As an athlete in high school, basketball was very important to me. Especially my senior year. We had a small school, and after years of practicing and training and taking a back seat to the older players, it was time to step up and lead our team (At least that is how I felt the great responsibility on my shoulders!).

We had already spent months with Pre-season practices (and the first third of the season, before Christmas) and I was playing well and stepping up as a leader on our team. It felt good, even though we were an "average" team, winning about half our games.

Over the Christmas holidays, I went with our Church on a "ski" trip to "Sugar Mountain" in North Carolina. On the last day of our trip (December 29th), on the last ski trip down the mountain, I decided to hit a "little" jump. I had been skiing well and enjoying myself, so I had become comfortable with taking small risks like that. Suffice it to say, I should never had taken that jump. When I returned to earth it was face first, and I actually landed straight on my shoulder.

I heard my collar bone snap like a twig.

After x-rays and a sling, I was headed back home on the bus. It was a clean break, and the pain was significant, but I was crying like a baby. Not because of the pain, but because I was going to let my team down by missing the rest of the basketball season.

"Life is so unfair" - was all I could think.

While visiting my regular physician back home, I pumped him for information on how fast I could recover, and how long it would take to get back in the game. I was tired of complaining and feeling like a bystander. I wanted to know what I could do to speed up the recovery process. He told me that there were some vitamin and nutritional procedures that looked promising, but that he was not very familiar with them. He scheduled a second visit about 10 days out (January 11th) for a follow-up, so that by then, he would know more about when I would be able to resume basketball.

I began researching immediately what I should do to speed up the bone repair process. My mother was an alternative therapy "junkie," so I had plenty of resources around the house. I started reading them ALL, looking for those nutritional therapies that might help me get better FAST.

Most of the information (even at that time) was unverified "propaganda" pitching different nutrition, but some of it had the sound of "truth." I made a plan from the most common nutritional therapies mentioned…. And my mother was more than happy to help me on my "Rapid Bone Repair" quest by purchasing the Bone Meal, the gelatin, the Fulvic Acid and the multivitamins that I needed in order to "attack" my broken collar bone.

So, I started a temporary "shock-load" treatment plan with multiple nutrients and vitamins. In the research, I had noticed that there were certain exercises and physical therapies that were recommended, so I started exercising in my sling.

The whole time I was doing this therapy, I was sitting on the sidelines watching "my" teammates practice, and they were preparing for an upcoming basketball tournament, beginning on January 12th.

Whether it was the shock-loading, or my general good health and youth, or the exercises I was doing…. I don't know. What I do know is that when we went back to the doctor on January the 11th for a checkup, I asked him when I would be able to play ball again. He examined me, worked with the collar bone, and then actually took an X-ray.

After looking at the X-ray for a while, he came in and said that, as far as he was concerned, I could start back playing basketball that evening. I had not told him about my "shock-loading". But after a full examination and an X-ray, he said, "go for it." He was VERY happy with the progress of the healing.

All in, from fracture (a complete fracture) to "competition ready" took exactly 14 days!

Again, this story is circumstantial and personal, I know, I know. It does not "prove" that others can be back on their feet as rapidly. It doesn't even technically "prove" anything, other than being a good story, (and one that I was glad to be a part of… at least the second half). I could have healed quickly, because I was young and active, or any number of other factors…But, what this experience did was make me aware that there are powerful nutritional forces that I knew little about….Even my doctor didn't know about these nutritional forces for healing either (at least at that time)!

That started my thirst for learning and researching about "health", about "recovery" and about the most rapid ways to repair broken bones. I have not stopped learning, and each time I break another bone (twice more), I would further refine my recipe and my "bone repair protocol."

I have shared this protocol with many friends over the years. Many look at me as if I am "slightly deranged." But, when and if they follow up on the protocol, they ALL thank me wholeheartedly.

And now it is time to share my personal experience, so that others might benefit. I know it is not "rock solid proof," but in conjunction with the actual clinical research that has been continuing for these past 30 years, there is now much more good clinical medical evidence that these nutritional therapies positively affect the rate of bone repair. Add those nutritional therapies with the physical therapy exercises and the other micro-movement therapies explained in the protocol, and there is a good reason to give it a shot. What is there to lose? Other than your "bystander," "helpless" and "victim" status?

OK, now to the end of the story. I did play in that tournament. I could not lift my right arm up over my head without a lot of pain, so I was essentially left handed. I scored 4 points. We got killed. The doctor was right. My collar bone was just fine, but I wasn't much help to the team.

Randy Velker

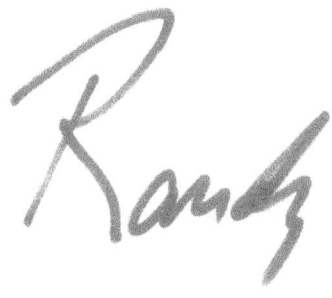

Appendix B

Bibliography

Aaseth, J., Boivin, G., & Andersen, O. (2012). Osteoporosis and trace elements–an overview. *Journal of Trace Elements in Medicine and Biology : Organ of the Society for Minerals and Trace Elements (GMS)*, *26*(2-3), 149–52. http://doi.org/10.1016/j.jtemb.2012.03.017

Agarwal, S. P., Khanna, R., Karmarkar, R., Anwer, M. K., & Khar, R. K. (2007). Shilajit: a review. *Phytotherapy Research*, *21*(5), 401–405. http://doi.org/10.1002/ptr.2100

Ahmadieh, H., & Arabi, A. (2011). Vitamins and bone health: beyond calcium and vitamin D. *Nutrition Reviews*, *69*(10), 584–98. http://doi.org/10.1111/j.1753-4887.2011.00372.x

Alcantara-Martos, T., Delgado-Martinez, A. D., Vega, M. V., Carrascal, M. T., Munuera-Martinez, L., & Surgeon, O. (2007). Effect of vitamin C on fracture healing in elderly Osteogenic Disorder Shionogi rats. *J Bone Joint Surg [Br]*, *89*, 402–7. http://doi.org/10.1302/0301-620X.89B3

Armas, L. A. G., Hollis, B. W., & Heaney, R. P. (2004). Vitamin D 2 Is Much Less Effective than Vitamin D 3 in Humans. *The Journal of Clinical Endocrinology & Metabolism*, *89*(11), 5387–5391. http://doi.org/10.1210/jc.2004-0360

Armstrong, T. A., & Spears, J. W. (2001). Effect of dietary boron on growth performance, calcium and phosphorus metabolism, and bone mechanical properties in growing barrows. *Journal of Animal Science*, *79*(12), 3120–7.

Avenell, A., & Handoll, H. H. (2010). Nutritional supplementation for hip fracture aftercare in older people. *The Cochrane Database of Systematic Reviews*, (1), CD001880. http://doi.org/10.1002/14651858.CD001880.pub5

Aydin, H., Deyneli, O., Yavuz, D., Gözü, H., Mutlu, N., Kaygusuz, I., & Akalin, S. (2010). Short-term oral magnesium supplementation suppresses bone turnover in postmenopausal osteoporotic women. *Biological Trace Element Research*, *133*(2), 136–43. http://doi.org/10.1007/s12011-009-8416-8

Azuma, K., Izumi, R., Osaki, T., Ifuku, S., Morimoto, M., Saimoto, H. … Okamoto, Y. (2015). Chitin, chitosan, and its derivatives for wound healing: old and new materials. *Journal of Functional Biomaterials*, *6*(1), 104–42. http://doi.org/10.3390/jfb6010104

Bae, Y.-J., & Kim, M.-H. (2008). Manganese supplementation improves mineral density of the spine and femur and serum osteocalcin in rats. *Biological Trace Element Research*, *124*(1), 28–34. http://doi.org/10.1007/s12011-008-8119-6

Barrio, D. A., & Etcheverry, S. B. (2006). Vanadium and bone development: putative signaling pathways. *Canadian Journal of Physiology and Pharmacology*, *84*(7), 677–86. http://doi.org/10.1139/y06-022

Barrio, D. A., & Etcheverry, S. B. (2010). Potential use of vanadium compounds in therapeutics. *Current Medicinal Chemistry*, *17*(31), 3632–42.

Bhattacharya, S. K., Sen, A. P., & Ghosal, S. (1995). Effects of shilajit on biogenic free radicals. *Phytotherapy Research*, *9*(1), 56–59. http://doi.org/10.1002/ptr.2650090113

Bonjour, J.-P. (2005). Dietary protein: an essential nutrient for bone health. *Journal of the American College of Nutrition*, *24*(6 Suppl.), 526S–36S.

Boskey, A. L., Wright, T. M., & Blank, R. D. (1999). Collagen and Bone Strength. *Journal of*

Bone and Mineral Research, *14*(3), 330–335. http://doi.org/10.1359/jbmr.1999.14.3.330

Cagno, V., Donalisio, M., Civra, A., Cagliero, C., Rubiolo, P., & Lembo, D. (2015). In vitro evaluation of the antiviral properties of Shilajit and investigation of its mechanisms of action. *Journal of Ethnopharmacology*, *166*, 129–34. http://doi.org/10.1016/j.jep.2015.03.019

Calvez, J., Poupin, N., Chesneau, C., Lassale, C., & Tomé, D. (2012). Protein intake, calcium balance and health consequences. *European Journal of Clinical Nutrition*, *66*(3), 281–95. http://doi.org/10.1038/ejcn.2011.196

Carlisle, E. M. (1970). Silicon: A Possible Factor in Bone Calcification. *Science*, *167*(3916), 279–280. http://doi.org/10.1126/science.167.3916.279

Carrasco-Gallardo, C., Farías, G. A., Fuentes, P., Crespo, F., & Maccioni, R. B. (2012). Can nutraceuticals prevent Alzheimer's disease? Potential therapeutic role of a formulation containing shilajit and complex B vitamins. *Archives of Medical Research*, *43*(8), 699–704. http://doi.org/10.1016/j.arcmed.2012.10.010

Carrasco-Gallardo, C., Guzmán, L., & Maccioni, R. B. (2012). Shilajit: a natural phytocomplex with potential procognitive activity. *International Journal of Alzheimer's Disease*, *2012*, 674142. http://doi.org/10.1155/2012/674142

Castelo-Branco, C., Ciria-Recasens, M., Cancelo-Hidalgo, M. J., Palacios, S., Haya-Palazuelos, J., Carbonell-Abelló, J. … Pérez-Edo, L. (n.d.). Efficacy of ossein-hydroxyapatite complex compared with calcium carbonate to prevent bone loss: a meta-analysis. *Menopause (New York, N.Y.)*, *16*(5), 984–91. http://doi.org/10.1097/gme.0b013e3181a1824e

Castelo-Branco, C., & Dávila Guardia, J. (2015). Use of ossein-hydroxyapatite complex in the prevention of bone loss: a review. *Climacteric : The Journal of the International Menopause Society*, *18*(1), 29–37. http://doi.org/10.3109/13697137.2014.929107

Chakkalakal, D. A., Novak, J. R., Fritz, E. D., Mollner, T. J., McVicker, D. L., Garvin, K. L., … Donohue, T. M. (2005). Inhibition of bone repair in a rat model for chronic and excessive alcohol consumption. *Alcohol (Fayetteville, N.Y.)*, *36*(3), 201–14. http://doi.org/10.1016/j.alcohol.2005.08.001

Chesnick, I. E., Todorov, T. I., Centeno, J. A., Newbury, D. E., Small, J. A., & Potter, K. (2007). Manganese-enhanced magnetic resonance microscopy of mineralization. *Magnetic Resonance Imaging*, *25*(7), 1095–104. http://doi.org/10.1016/j.mri.2006.11.002

Chevrier, A., Hoemann, C. D., Sun, J., & Buschmann, M. D. (2007). Chitosan-glycerol phosphate/blood implants increase cell recruitment, transient vascularization and subchondral bone remodeling in drilled cartilage defects. *Osteoarthritis and Cartilage / OARS, Osteoarthritis Research Society*, *15*(3), 316–27. http://doi.org/10.1016/j.joca.2006.08.007

Claes, L., Eckert-Hübner, K., & Augat, P. (2002). The effect of mechanical stability on local vascularization and tissue differentiation in callus healing. *Journal of Orthopaedic Research : Official Publication of the Orthopaedic Research Society*, *20*(5), 1099–105. http://doi.org/10.1016/S0736-0266 (02)00044-X

Claes, L., & Willie, B. (n.d.). The enhancement of bone regeneration by ultrasound. *Progress in Biophysics and Molecular Biology*, *93*(1-3), 384–98. http://doi.org/10.1016/j.pbiomolbio.2006.07.021

Cook, J. J., Summers, N. J., & Cook, E. A. (2015). Healing in the new millennium: bone stimulators: an overview of where we've been and where we may be heading. *Clinics in Podiatric Medicine and Surgery*, *32*(1), 45–59. http://doi.org/10.1016/j.cpm.2014.09.003

Cranney, A., Horsley, T., O'Donnell, S., Weiler, H., Puil, L., Ooi, D. … Mamaladze, V. (2007). Effectiveness and safety of vitamin D in relation to bone health. *Evidence Report/technology Assessment*, (158), 1–235.

Cusack, P. (2008). Effects of a dietary complex of humic and fulvic acids (FeedMAX 15^{TM})

on the health and production of feedlot cattle destined for the Australian domestic market. *Australian Veterinary Journal, 86*(1-2), 46–49. http://doi.org/10.1111/j.1751-0813.2007.00242.x

Cusack, P. M. V. (n.d.). Effects of a dietary complex of humic and fulvic acids (FeedMAX 15) on the health and production of feedlot cattle destined for the Australian domestic market. *Australian Veterinary Journal, 86*(1-2), 46–9. http://doi.org/10.1111/j.1751-0813.2007.00242.x

Dai, Z., & Koh, W.-P. (2015). B-Vitamins and Bone Health–A Review of the Current Evidence. *Nutrients, 7*(5), 3322–3346. http://doi.org/10.3390/nu7053322

Devrimsel, G., Turkyilmaz, A. K., Yildirim, M., & Beyazal, M. S. (2015). The effects of whirlpool bath and neuromuscular electrical stimulation on complex regional pain syndrome. *Journal of Physical Therapy Science, 27*(1), 27–30. http://doi.org/10.1589/jpts.27.27

Dimai, H.-P. (1998). Daily Oral Magnesium Supplementation Suppresses Bone Turnover in Young Adult Males. *Journal of Clinical Endocrinology & Metabolism, 83*(8), 2742–2748. http://doi.org/10.1210/jc.83.8.2742

D'Mello, S., Elangovan, S., Hong, L., Ross, R. D., Sumner, D. R., & Salem, A. K. (2015). Incorporation of copper into chitosan scaffolds promotes bone regeneration in rat calvarial defects. *Journal of Biomedical Materials Research. Part B, Applied Biomaterials, 103*(5), 1044–9. http://doi.org/10.1002/jbm.b.33290

Dodds, R. A., Catterall, A., Bitensky, L., & Chayen, J. (1986). Abnormalities in fracture healing induced by vitamin B6-deficiency in rats. *Bone, 7*(6), 489–495. http://doi.org/10.1016/8756-3282 (86)90008-6

Einhorn, T. A., Bonnarens, F., & Burstein, A. H. (1986). The contributions of dietary protein and mineral to the healing of experimental fractures. A biomechanical study. *J Bone Joint Surg Am, 68*(9), 1389–1395.

Einhorn, T. A., & Gerstenfeld, L. C. (2015). Fracture healing: mechanisms and interventions. *Nature Reviews. Rheumatology, 11*(1), 45–54. http://doi.org/10.1038/nrrheum.2014.164

Epari, D. R., Kassi, J.-P., Schell, H., & Duda, G. N. (2007). Timely fracture-healing requires optimization of axial fixation stability. *The Journal of Bone and Joint Surgery. American Volume, 89*(7), 1575–85. http://doi.org/10.2106/JBJS.F.00247

Everson, C. A., Folley, A. E., & Toth, J. M. (2012). Chronically inadequate sleep results in abnormal bone formation and abnormal bone marrow in rats. *Experimental Biology and Medicine, 237*(9), 1101–1109. http://doi.org/10.1258/ebm.2012.012043

Ezoddini-Ardakani, F., Navabazam, A., Fatehi, F., Danesh-Ardekani, M., Khadem, S., & Rouhi, G. (2012). Histologic evaluation of chitosan as an accelerator of bone regeneration in microdrilled rat tibias. *Dental Research Journal, 9*(6), 694–9.

Ezoddini-Ardakani, F., Navab Azam, A., Yassaei, S., Fatehi, F., & Rouhi, G. (2011). Effects of chitosan on dental bone repair. *Health, 03*(04), 200–205. http://doi.org/10.4236/health.2011.34036

Figueres Juher, T., & Basés Pérez, E. (2015). Revisión de los efectos beneficiosos de la ingesta de colágeno hidrolizado sobre la salud osteoarticular y el envejecimiento dérmico AN OVERVIEW OF THE BENEFICIAL EFFECTS OF HYDROLYSED COLLAGEN INTAKE ON JOINT AND BONE HEALTH AND ON SKIN AGEING. *Nutr Hosp.Nutr Hosp, 3232*(1), 62–6662. http://doi.org/10.3305/nh.2015.32.sup1.9482

Fujii, K., Kajiwara, T., & Kurosu, H. (1979). Effect of vitamin B6 deficiency on the crosslink formation of collagen. *FEBS Letters, 97*(1), 193–195. http://doi.org/10.1016/0014-5793 (79)80082-4

Gandy, J. (2012). Phase 1 clinical study of the acute and subacute safety and proof-of-concept efficacy of carbohydrate-derived fulvic acid. *Clinical Pharmacology: Advances and Applications, 7*. http://doi.org/10.2147/CPAA.S25784

Ganta, D. R., McCarthy, M.-B., & Gronowicz, G. A. (1997). Ascorbic Acid Alters Collagen

Integrins in Bone Culture [1]. *Endocrinology*, *138*(9), 3606–3612. http://doi.org/10.1210/endo.138.9.5367

Gardner, M. J., Putnam, S. M., Wong, A., Streubel, P. N., Kotiya, A., & Silva, M. J. (2011). Differential fracture healing resulting from fixation stiffness variability: a mouse model. *Journal of Orthopaedic Science*, *16*(3), 298–303. http://doi.org/10.1007/s00776-011-0051-5

Genuis, S. J., & Bouchard, T. P. (2012). Combination of Micronutrients for Bone (COMB) Study: bone density after micronutrient intervention. *Journal of Environmental and Public Health*, *2012*, 354151. http://doi.org/10.1155/2012/354151

Gigante, A., Torcianti, M., Boldrini, E., Manzotti, S., Falcone, G., Greco, F., & Mattioli-Belmonte, M. (n.d.). Vitamin K and D association stimulates in vitro osteoblast differentiation of fracture site derived human mesenchymal stem cells. *Journal of Biological Regulators and Homeostatic Agents*, *22*(1), 35–44.

Gong, T., Xie, J., Liao, J., Zhang, T., Lin, S., & Lin, Y. (2015). Nanomaterials and bone regeneration. *Bone Research*, *3*, 15029. http://doi.org/10.1038/boneres.2015.29

Goodship, A., & Kenwright, J. (1985). The influence of induced micro movement upon the healing of experimental tibial fractures. *Bone & Joint Journal*, *67-B* (4), 650–655.

Gouin, J.-P., & Kiecolt-Glaser, J. K. (2011). The Impact of Psychological Stress on Wound Healing: Methods and Mechanisms. *Immunology and Allergy Clinics of North America*, *31*(1), 81–93. http://doi.org/10.1016/j.iac.2010.09.010

Grosso, G., Bei, R., Mistretta, A., Marventano, S., Calabrese, G., Masuelli, L. … Gazzolo, D. (2013). Effects of vitamin C on health: a review of evidence. *Frontiers in Bioscience (Landmark Edition)*, *18*, 1017–29.

Gümüştekín, K., Seven, B., Karabulut, N., Aktaş, O., Gürsan, N., Aslan, S. … Dane, S. (2004). Effects of sleep deprivation, nicotine, and selenium on wound healing in rats. *The International Journal of Neuroscience*, *114*(11), 1433–42.

Guralp, O., & Erel, C. T. (2014). Effects of vitamin K in postmenopausal women: mini review. *Maturitas*, *77*(3), 294–9. http://doi.org/10.1016/j.maturitas.2013.11.002

Haramizu, S., Ota, N., Hase, T., & Murase, T. (2013). Catechins suppress muscle inflammation and hasten performance recovery after exercise. *Medicine and Science in Sports and Exercise*, *45*(9), 1694–702. http://doi.org/10.1249/MSS.0b013e31828de99f

Heaney, R. P., Abrams, S., Dawson-Hughes, B., Looker, A., Looker, A., Marcus, R. … Weaver, C. (2001). Peak Bone Mass. *Osteoporosis International*, *11*(12), 985–1009. http://doi.org/10.1007/s001980070020

Heaney, R. P., & Weaver, C. M. (2005). Newer Perspectives on Calcium Nutrition and Bone Quality. *Journal of the American College of Nutrition*, *24*(sup6), 574S–581S. http://doi.org/10.1080/07315724.2005.10719506

Hinton, P. S., Nigh, P., & Thyfault, J. (2015). Effectiveness of resistance training or jumping-exercise to increase bone mineral density in men with low bone mass: A 12-month randomized, clinical trial. *Bone*, *79*, 203–212. http://doi.org/10.1016/j.bone.2015.06.008

Holick, M. F. (2006). High Prevalence of Vitamin D Inadequacy and Implications for Health. *Mayo Clinic Proceedings*, *81*(3), 353–373. http://doi.org/10.4065/81.3.353

Hoogendoorn, J. M., Simmermacher, R. K. J., Schellekens, P. P. A., & van der Werken, C. (2002). [Adverse effects of smoking on healing of bones and soft tissues]. *Der Unfallchirurg*, *105*(1), 76–81.

Hreha, J., Wey, A., Cunningham, C., Krell, E. S., Brietbart, E. A., Paglia, D. N., … Lin, S. S. (2015). Local manganese chloride treatment accelerates fracture healing in a rat model. *Journal of Orthopaedic Research : Official Publication of the Orthopaedic Research Society*, *33*(1), 122–30. http://doi.org/10.1002/jor.22733

Igarashi, A., & Yamaguchi, M. (2003). Great increase in bone 66 kDa protein and osteocalcin at later stages with healing rat fractures: effect of zinc treatment. *International Journal of*

Molecular Medicine, *11*(2), 223–8.

Inaba, N., Sato, T., & Yamashita, T. (2015). Low-Dose Daily Intake of Vitamin K2 (Menaquinone-7) Improves Osteocalcin γ-Carboxylation: A Double-Blind, Randomized Controlled Trials. *Journal of Nutritional Science and Vitaminology*, *61*(6), 471–80. http://doi.org/10.3177/jnsv.61.471

Ishimi, Y. (2010). [Nutrition and bone health. Magnesium and bone]. *Clinical Calcium*, *20*(5), 762–7. http://doi.org/CliCa1005762767

Islam, K. M. S., Schaeublin, H., Wenk, C., Wanner, M., & Liesegang, A. (2012). Effect of dietary citric acid on the performance and mineral metabolism of broiler. *Journal of Animal Physiology and Animal Nutrition*, *96*(5), 808–817. http://doi.org/10.1111/j.1439-0396.2011.01225.x

Jagodzinski, M., & Krettek, C. (2007). Effect of mechanical stability on fracture healing–an update. *Injury*, *38 Suppl 1*, S3–10. http://doi.org/10.1016/j.injury.2007.02.005

Jaiswal, A. K., & Bhattacharya, S. K. (1992). Effect of Shilajit on memory, anxiety and brain monoamines in rats. *Indian Journal of Pharmacology*, *24*.

Jingushi, S. (2009). [Bone fracture and the healing mechanisms. Fracture treatment by low-intensity pulsed ultrasound]. *Clinical Calcium*, *19*(5), 704–8. http://doi.org/CliCa0905704708

Jugdaohsingh, R. (n.d.). SILICON AND BONE HEALTH.

Jugdaohsingh, R., Tucker, K. L., Qiao, N., Cupples, L. A., Kiel, D. P., & Powell, J. J. (2003). Dietary Silicon Intake Is Positively Associated With Bone Mineral Density in Men and Premenopausal Women of the Framingham Offspring Cohort. *Journal of Bone and Mineral Research*, *19*(2), 297–307. http://doi.org/10.1359/JBMR.0301225

Kang, S.-H., & Choi, W. (2009). Oxidative degradation of organic compounds using zero-valent iron in the presence of natural organic matter serving as an electron shuttle. *Environmental Science & Technology*, *43*(3), 878–83.

Kasturi, G., & Adler, R. A. (2011). Mechanical means to improve bone strength: ultrasound and vibration. *Current Rheumatology Reports*, *13*(3), 251–6. http://doi.org/10.1007/s11926-011-0177-7

Knapen, M. H. J. (1989). The Effect of Vitamin K Supplementation on Circulating Osteocalcin (Bone Gla Protein) and Urinary Calcium Excretion. *Annals of Internal Medicine*, *111*(12), 1001. http://doi.org/10.7326/0003-4819-111-12-1001

Koitaya, N., Sekiguchi, M., Tousen, Y., Nishide, Y., Morita, A., Yamauchi, J. … Ishimi, Y. (2014). Low-dose vitamin K2 (MK-4) supplementation for 12 months improves bone metabolism and prevents forearm bone loss in postmenopausal Japanese women. *Journal of Bone and Mineral Metabolism*, *32*(2), 142–150. http://doi.org/10.1007/s00774-013-0472-7

Liem, A., Pesti, G. M., & Edwards, H. M. (2008). The Effect of Several Organic Acids on Phytate Phosphorus Hydrolysis in Broiler Chicks. *Poultry Science*, *87*(4), 689–693. http://doi.org/10.3382/ps.2007-00256

Li, J., Yuan, J., Guo, Y., Sun, Q., & Hu, X. (2012). The Influence of Dietary Calcium and Phosphorus Imbalance on Intestinal NaPi-IIb and Calbindin mRNA Expression and Tibia Parameters of Broilers. *Asian-Australasian Journal of Animal Sciences*, *25*(4), 552–558. http://doi.org/10.5713/ajas.2011.11266

Liu, H., Li, H., Cheng, W., Yang, Y., Zhu, M., & Zhou, C. (2006). Novel injectable calcium phosphate/chitosan composites for bone substitute materials. *Acta Biomaterialia*, *2*(5), 557–565. http://doi.org/10.1016/j.actbio.2006.03.007

Liu, P.-Y., Brummel-Smith, K., & Ilich, J. Z. (2011). Aerobic Exercise and Whole-Body Vibration in Offsetting Bone Loss in Older Adults. *SAGE-Hindawi Access to Research Journal of Aging Research*, *379674*. http://doi.org/10.4061/2011/379674

Li, Y., & Stahl, C. H. (2014). Dietary Calcium Deficiency and Excess Both Impact Bone Development and Mesenchymal Stem Cell Lineage Priming in Neonatal Piglets. *Journal of Nutrition*, *144*(12), 1935–1942. http://doi.org/10.3945/jn.114.194787

Maatoq Hashim, A. (2014). JOURNAL OF INTERNATIONAL ACADEMIC RESEARCH FOR MULTIDISCIPLINARY RADIOLOGICAL AND HISTOPATHOLOGICAL STUDY OF THE EFFECTIVENESS THE NON-STEROIDAL ANTI-INFLAMMATORY DRUG ON THE HEALING OF FRACTURE IN RABBITS, *2*(11), 2320–5083.

Mackay, D., & Miller, A. L. (2003). Nutritional Support for Wound Healing. *Alternative Medicine Review* ◆, *8*(4).

Mahajan, A., Alexander, L. S., Seabolt, B. S., Catrambone, D. E., McClung, J. P., Odle, J., … Stahl, C. H. (2011). Dietary Calcium Restriction Affects Mesenchymal Stem Cell Activity and Bone Development in Neonatal Pigs. *Journal of Nutrition*, *141*(3), 373–379. http://doi.org/10.3945/jn.110.131193

Mahdavi-Roshan, M., Ebrahimi, M., & Ebrahimi, A. (n.d.). Copper, magnesium, zinc and calcium status in osteopenic and osteoporotic post-menopausal women. *Clinical Cases in Mineral and Bone Metabolism : The Official Journal of the Italian Society of Osteoporosis, Mineral Metabolism, and Skeletal Diseases*, *12*(1), 18–21. http://doi.org/10.11138/ccmbm/2015.12.1.018

Manganese deficiency associated with bone deformities in calves. (2013). *The Veterinary Record*, *172*(15), 389–92. http://doi.org/10.1136/vr.f2024

Mathuthu, A. S., & Ephraim, J. H. (1993). Calcium binding by fulvic acids studied by an ion selective electrode an ultrafiltration method. *Talanta*, *40*(4), 521–526. http://doi.org/10.1016/0039-9140 (93)80011-F

McCoy, H., Kenney, M. A., Montgomery, C., Irwin, A., Williams, L., & Orrell, R. (1994). Relation of Boron to the Composition and Mechanical Properties of Bone. *Environmental Health Perspectives*, *102*, 49. http://doi.org/10.2307/3431962

Moores, J. (2013). Vitamin C: a wound healing perspective. *British Journal of Community Nursing*, *Suppl*, S6, S8–11.

Mooventhan, A., & Nivethitha, L. (2014). Scientific evidence-based effects of hydrotherapy on various systems of the body. *North American Journal of Medical Sciences*, *6*(5), 199–209. http://doi.org/10.4103/1947-2714.132935

Mundi, R., Petis, S., Kaloty, R., Shetty, V., & Bhandari, M. (2009). Low-intensity pulsed ultrasound: Fracture healing. *Indian Journal of Orthopaedics*, *43*(2), 132–40. http://doi.org/10.4103/0019-5413.50847

Nakaya, Y., Uehara, M., Katsumata, S.-I., Suzuki, K., Sakai, K., Ohnishi, R. … Ohta, A. (2010). The frequency of magnesium consumption directly influences its serum concentration and the amount of elutable bone magnesium in rats. *Magnesium Research : Official Organ of the International Society for the Development of Research on Magnesium*, *23*(1), 48–56. http://doi.org/10.1684/mrh.2009.0197

Nash, L. A., & Ward, W. E. (2015). Tea and Bone Health: Findings from Human Studies, Potential Mechanisms, and Identification of Knowledge Gaps. *Critical Reviews in Food Science and Nutrition*, 00–00. http://doi.org/10.1080/10408398.2014.1001019

Nikander, R., Sievänen, H., Heinonen, A., Daly, R. M., Uusi-Rasi, K., & Kannus, P. (2010). Targeted exercise against osteoporosis: A systematic review and meta-analysis for optimising bone strength throughout life. *BMC Medicine*, *8*(1), 47. http://doi.org/10.1186/1741-7015-8-47

O'Daly, B. J., Walsh, J. C., Quinlan, J. F., Falk, G. A., Stapleton, R., Quinlan, W. R., & O'Rourke, S. K. (2010). Serum albumin and total lymphocyte count as predictors of outcome in hip fractures. *Clinical Nutrition (Edinburgh, Scotland)*, *29*(1), 89–93. http://doi.org/10.1016/j.clnu.2009.07.007

Oliveira, T. F. B., Bertechini, A. G., Bricka, R. M., Hester, P. Y., Kim, E. J., Gerard, P. D., & Peebles, E. D. (2015). Effects of in ovo injection of organic trace minerals and post-hatch holding time on broiler performance and bone characteristics. *Poultry Science, 94*(11), 2677–85. http://doi.org/10.3382/ps/pev249

Oyen, J., Apalset, E. M., Gjesdal, C. G., Brudvik, C., Lie, S. A., & Hove, L. M. (2011). Vitamin D inadequacy is associated with low-energy distal radius fractures: a case-control study. *Bone, 48*(5), 1140–5. http://doi.org/10.1016/j.bone.2011.01.021

Paglia, D. N., Wey, A., Park, A. G., Breitbart, E. A., Mehta, S. K., Bogden, J. D., … Lin, S. S. (2012). The effects of local vanadium treatment on angiogenesis and chondrogenesis during fracture healing. *Journal of Orthopaedic Research : Official Publication of the Orthopaedic Research Society, 30*(12), 1971–8. http://doi.org/10.1002/jor.22159

Palacios, C. (2006). The role of nutrients in bone health, from A to Z. *Critical Reviews in Food Science and Nutrition, 46*(8), 621–8. http://doi.org/10.1080/10408390500466174

Palomares, K. T. S., Gleason, R. E., Mason, Z. D., Cullinane, D. M., Einhorn, T. A., Gerstenfeld, L. C., & Morgan, E. F. (2009). Mechanical stimulation alters tissue differentiation and molecular expression during bone healing. *Journal of Orthopaedic Research, 27*(9), 1123–1132. http://doi.org/10.1002/jor.20863

Park, J.-S., Kim, G.-Y., & Han, K. (2006). The spermatogenic and ovogenic effects of chronically administered Shilajit to rats. *Journal of Ethnopharmacology, 107*(3), 349–53. http://doi.org/10.1016/j.jep.2006.03.039

Patel, R. A., Wilson, R. F., Patel, P. A., & Palmer, R. M. (2013). The effect of smoking on bone healing: A systematic review. *Bone and Joint Research, 2*(6), 102–111. http://doi.org/10.1302/2046-3758.26.2000142

Peacock, M. (2010). Calcium Metabolism in Health and Disease. *Clinical Journal of the American Society of Nephrology, 5*(Supplement 1), S23–S30. http://doi.org/10.2215/CJN.05910809

Persson, M., Hytter-Landahl, A., Brismar, K., & Cederholm, T. (2007). Nutritional supplementation and dietary advice in geriatric patients at risk of malnutrition. *Clinical Nutrition (Edinburgh, Scotland), 26*(2), 216–24. http://doi.org/10.1016/j.clnu.2006.12.002

Pizzorno, L. (2015). Nothing Boring About Boron. *Integrative Medicine (Encinitas, Calif.), 14*(4), 35–48.

Price, C. T., Koval, K. J., & Langford, J. R. (2013). Silicon: a review of its potential role in the prevention and treatment of postmenopausal osteoporosis. *International Journal of Endocrinology, 2013*, 316783. http://doi.org/10.1155/2013/316783

Price, C. T., Langford, J. R., & Liporace, F. A. (2012). Essential Nutrients for Bone Health and a Review of their Availability in the Average North American Diet. *The Open Orthopaedics Journal, 6*, 143–9. http://doi.org/10.2174/1874325001206010143

R, C., DT, V., D, A., P, N., LV, A., & C, G. (1991). Dietary L-lysine and calcium metabolism in humans. *Nutrition (Burbank, Los Angeles County, Calif.), 8*(6), 400–405.

Rector, R. S., Rogers, R., Ruebel, M., Widzer, M. O., & Hinton, P. S. (2009). Lean body mass and weight-bearing activity in the prediction of bone mineral density in physically active men. *Journal of Strength and Conditioning Research / National Strength & Conditioning Association, 23*(2), 427–35. http://doi.org/10.1519/JSC.0b013e31819420e1

Reid, D. M., & New, S. A. (1997). Nutritional influences on bone mass. *Proceedings of the Nutrition Society, 56*(03), 977–987. http://doi.org/10.1079/PNS19970103

Reid, I. R., & Bolland, M. J. (2008). Calcium supplementation and vascular disease. *Climacteric, 11*(4), 280–286. http://doi.org/10.1080/13697130802229639

Rondanelli, M., Opizzi, A., Perna, S., & Faliva, M. A. (2013). Update on nutrients involved in maintaining healthy bone. *Endocrinología Y Nutrición : órgano de La Sociedad Española de Endocrinología Y Nutrición, 60*(4), 197–210. http://doi.org/10.1016/j.endonu.2012.09.006

Rude, R. K., Gruber, H. E., Norton, H. J., Wei, L. Y., Frausto, A., & Kilburn, J. (2006). Reduction of dietary magnesium by only 50% in the rat disrupts bone and mineral metabolism. *Osteoporosis International : A Journal Established as Result of Cooperation between the European Foundation for Osteoporosis and the National Osteoporosis Foundation of the USA, 17*(7), 1022–32. http://doi.org/10.1007/s00198-006-0104-3

Rude, R. K., Singer, F. R., & Gruber, H. E. (2009). Skeletal and hormonal effects of magnesium deficiency. *Journal of the American College of Nutrition, 28*(2), 131–41.

Ryan-Harshman, M., & Aldoori, W. (2004). Bone health. New role for vitamin K? *Canadian Family Physician Médecin de Famille Canadien, 50*, 993–7.

Sacco, S. M., Horcajada, M.-N., & Offord, E. (2013). Phytonutrients for bone health during ageing. *British Journal of Clinical Pharmacology, 75*(3), 697–707. http://doi.org/10.1111/bcp.12033

Samira, J., Saoudi, M., Abdelmajid, K., Hassane, O., Treq, R., Hafed, E. … Hassib, K. (2015). Accelerated bone ingrowth by local delivery of Zinc from bioactive glass: oxidative stress status, mechanical property, and micro architectural characterization in an ovariectomized rat model. *The Libyan Journal of Medicine, 10*, 28572.

Sanchez, A., Reeser, J. L., Lau, H. S., Yahiku, P. Y., Willard, R. E., McMillan, P. J., … Register, U. D. (1973). Role of sugars in human neutrophilic phagocytosis. *The American Journal of Clinical Nutrition, 26*(11), 1180–1184.

Sanmanee, N., & Areekijseree, M. (2010). The effects of fulvic acid on copper bioavailability to porcine oviductal epithelial cells. *Biological Trace Element Research, 135*(1-3), 162–73. http://doi.org/10.1007/s12011-009-8508-5

Sato, T., Schurgers, L. J., & Uenishi, K. (2012). Comparison of menaquinone-4 and menaquinone-7 bioavailability in healthy women. *Nutrition Journal, 11*(1), 93. http://doi.org/10.1186/1475-2891-11-93

S. Chan, B. Gerson, S. S. (1998). The role of copper, molybdenum, selenium, and zinc in nutrition and health. *Clin Lab Med., 18(4)*, 673–685.

Schepetkin, I. A., Khlebnikov, A. I., Ah, S. Y., Woo, S. B., Jeong, C.-S., Klubachuk, O. N., & Kwon, B. S. (2003). Characterization and biological activities of humic substances from mumie. *Journal of Agricultural and Food Chemistry, 51*(18), 5245–54. http://doi.org/10.1021/jf021101e

Schepetkin, I. A., Xie, G., Jutila, M. A., & Quinn, M. T. (2009). Complement-fixing activity of fulvic acid from Shilajit and other natural sources. *Phytotherapy Research, 23*(3), 373–384. http://doi.org/10.1002/ptr.2635

Schepetkin, I., Khlebnikov, A., & Kwon, B. S. (2002). Medical drugs from humus matter: Focus on mumie. *Drug Development Research, 57*(3), 140–159. http://doi.org/10.1002/ddr.10058

Schmitz, M. A., Finnegan, M., Natarajan, R., & Champine, J. (1999). Effect of smoking on tibial shaft fracture healing. *Clinical Orthopaedics and Related Research*, (365), 184–200.

Shen, C.-L., Chyu, M.-C., & Wang, J.-S. (2013). Tea and bone health: steps forward in translational nutrition. *American Journal of Clinical Nutrition, 98*(6), 1694S–1699S. http://doi.org/10.3945/ajcn.113.058255

Shen, C.-L., Chyu, M.-C., Yeh, J. K., Zhang, Y., Pence, B. C., Felton, C. K., … Wang, J.-S. (2012). Effect of green tea and Tai Chi on bone health in postmenopausal osteopenic women: a 6-month randomized placebo-controlled trial. *Osteoporosis International, 23*(5), 1541–1552. http://doi.org/10.1007/s00198-011-1731-x

Sherry, L., Millhouse, E., Lappin, D. F., Murray, C., Culshaw, S., Nile, C. J., & Ramage, G. (2013). Investigating the biological properties of carbohydrate derived fulvic acid (CHD-FA) as a potential novel therapy for the management of oral biofilm infections. *BMC Oral Health, 13*, 47. http://doi.org/10.1186/1472-6831-13-47

Simşek, A., Senköylü, A., Cila, E., Uğurlu, M., Bayar, A., Oztürk, A. M. … Yetkin, H. (2006). [Is there a correlation between severity of trauma and serum trace element levels?]. *Acta Orthopaedica et Traumatologica Turcica, 40*(2), 140–3.

Song, H.-Y., Esfakur Rahman, A. H. M., & Lee, B.-T. (2009). Fabrication of calcium phosphate-calcium sulfate injectable bone substitute using chitosan and citric acid.

Journal of Materials Science: Materials in Medicine, 20(4), 935–941. http://doi.org/10.1007/s10856-008-3642-8

Spector, T. D., Calomme, M. R., Anderson, S. H., Clement, G., Bevan, L., Demeester, N. … Powell, J. J. (2008). Choline-stabilized orthosilicic acid supplementation as an adjunct to Calcium/Vitamin D3 stimulates markers of bone formation in osteopenic females: a randomized, placebo-controlled trial. *BMC Musculoskeletal Disorders, 9*(1), 85. http://doi.org/10.1186/1471-2474-9-85

Srivastava, S., Kumar, N., & Roy, P. (2014). Role of ERK/NFκB in vanadium (IV) oxide mediated osteoblast differentiation in C3H10t1/2 cells. *Biochimie, 101*, 132–44. http://doi.org/10.1016/j.biochi.2014.01.005

Srivastava, S., Kumar, N., Thakur, R. S., & Roy, P. (2013). Role of vanadium (V) in the differentiation of C3H10t1/2 cells towards osteoblast lineage: a comparative analysis with other trace elements. *Biological Trace Element Research, 152*(1), 135–42. http://doi.org/10.1007/s12011-013-9602-2

Stohs, S. J. (2014). Safety and efficacy of shilajit (mumie, moomiyo). *Phytotherapy Research : PTR, 28*(4), 475–9. http://doi.org/10.1002/ptr.5018

Surapaneni, D. K., Adapa, S. R. S. S., Preeti, K., Teja, G. R., Veeraragavan, M., & Krishnamurthy, S. (2012). Shilajit attenuates behavioral symptoms of chronic fatigue syndrome by modulating the hypothalamic-pituitary-adrenal axis and mitochondrial bioenergetics in rats. *Journal of Ethnopharmacology, 143*(1), 91–9. http://doi.org/10.1016/j.jep.2012.06.002

Tang, B. M., Eslick, G. D., Nowson, C., Smith, C., & Bensoussan, A. (2007). Use of calcium or calcium in combination with vitamin D supplementation to prevent fractures and bone loss in people aged 50 years and older: a meta-analysis. *The Lancet, 370*(9588), 657–666. http://doi.org/10.1016/S0140-6736 (07)61342-7

Tarafder, S., Davies, N. M., Bandyopadhyay, A., & Bose, S. (2013). 3D printed tricalcium phosphate scaffolds: Effect of SrO and MgO doping on in vivo osteogenesis in a rat distal femoral defect model. *Biomaterials Science, 1*(12), 1250–1259. http://doi.org/10.1039/C3BM60132C

Traber, M. G., & Stevens, J. F. (2011). Vitamins C and E: Beneficial effects from a mechanistic perspective. *Free Radical Biology and Medicine, 51*(5), 1000–1013. http://doi.org/10.1016/j.freeradbiomed.2011.05.017

Trautvetter, U., Jahreis, G., Kiehntopf, M., & Glei, M. (2016). Consequences of a high phosphorus intake on mineral metabolism and bone remodeling in dependence of calcium intake in healthy subjects - a randomized placebo-controlled human intervention study. *Nutrition Journal, 15*(1), 7. http://doi.org/10.1186/s12937-016-0125-5

Trautvetter, U., Neef, N., Leiterer, M., Kiehntopf, M., Kratzsch, J., & Jahreis, G. (2014). Effect of calcium phosphate and vitamin D3 supplementation on bone remodelling and metabolism of calcium, phosphorus, magnesium and iron. *Nutrition Journal, 13*(1), 6. http://doi.org/10.1186/1475-2891-13-6

van Rensburg, C. E. J. (2015). The Anti-inflammatory Properties of Humic Substances: A Mini Review. *Phytotherapy Research, 29*(6), 791–795. http://doi.org/10.1002/ptr.5319

Vedakumari, W. S., Prabu, P., & Sastry, T. P. (2015). Chitosan-Fibrin Nanocomposites as Drug Delivering and Wound Healing Materials. *Journal of Biomedical Nanotechnology, 11*(4), 657–67.

Verma, S., Singh, A., & Mishra, A. (2013). The effect of fulvic acid on pre- and post-aggregation state of Aβ (17-42): molecular dynamics simulation studies. *Biochimica et Biophysica Acta, 1834*(1), 24–33. http://doi.org/10.1016/j.bbapap.2012.08.016

Victoria, G., Petrisor, B., Drew, B., & Dick, D. (2009). Bone stimulation for fracture healing: What's all the fuss? *Indian Journal of Orthopaedics, 43*(2), 117–20. http://doi.org/10.4103/0019-5413.50844

Viguet-Carrin, S., Garnero, P., & Delmas, P. D. (2006). The role of collagen in bone strength.

Osteoporosis International, *17*(3), 319–336. http://doi.org/10.1007/s00198-005-2035-9

Vucskits, A. V., Hullár, I., Bersényi, A., Andrásofszky, E., Kulcsár, M., & Szabó, J. (2010). Effect of fulvic and humic acids on performance, immune response and thyroid function in rats. *Journal of Animal Physiology and Animal Nutrition*, *94*(6), 721–8. http://doi.org/10.1111/j.1439-0396.2010.01023.x

Walker, A. F., Marakis, G., Christie, S., & Byng, M. (2003). Mg citrate found more bioavailable than other Mg preparations in a randomised, double-blind study. *Magnesium Research : Official Organ of the International Society for the Development of Research on Magnesium*, *16*(3), 183–91.

Wang, G., Wang, J., Fu, Y., Bai, L., He, M., Li, B., & Fu, Q. (2013). Systemic treatment with vanadium absorbed by Coprinus comatus promotes femoral fracture healing in streptozotocin-diabetic rats. *Biological Trace Element Research*, *151*(3), 424–33. http://doi.org/10.1007/s12011-012-9584-5

Watanabe, Y., Matsushita, T., Bhandari, M., Zdero, R., & Schemitsch, E. H. (2010). Ultrasound for fracture healing: current evidence. *Journal of Orthopaedic Trauma*, *24 Suppl 1*, S56–61. http://doi.org/10.1097/BOT.0b013e3181d2efaf

White, S. H., Cunningham, J. L., Richardson, J. B., Evans, M., Kenwright, J., Adams, M. A. … Newman, J. H. (1991). Improvement of Fracture Healing by Applied Axial Micromovement: A Clinical Study. In *Interfaces in Medicine and Mechanics—2* (pp. 243–248). Dordrecht: Springer Netherlands. Retrieved from http://www.springerlink.com/index/10.1007/978-94-011-3852-9_24

Yamada, P., Isoda, H., Kyu HAN, J., N Talorete, T. P., Yamaguchi, T., & Abe, Y. (n.d.). Inhibitory Effect of Fulvic Acid Extracted from Canadian Sphagnum Peat on Chemical Mediator Release by RBL-2H3 and KU812 Cells. http://doi.org/10.1271/bbb.60702

Yamaguchi, M. (2010). Role of nutritional zinc in the prevention of osteoporosis. *Molecular and Cellular Biochemistry*, *338*(1-2), 241–54. http://doi.org/10.1007/s11010-009-0358-0

Yamaguchi, M. (2012). Nutritional factors and bone homeostasis: synergistic effect with zinc and genistein in osteogenesis. *Molecular and Cellular Biochemistry*, *366*(1-2), 201–21. http://doi.org/10.1007/s11010-012-1298-7

Yamamoto, S., & Uenishi, K. (2010). [Nutrition and bone health. Magnesium-rich foods and bone health]. *Clinical Calcium*, *20*(5), 768–74. http://doi.org/CliCa1005768774

Yuasa, M., Mignemi, N. A., Nyman, J. S., Duvall, C. L., Schwartz, H. S., Okawa, A., … Schoenecker, J. G. (2015). Fibrinolysis is essential for fracture repair and prevention of heterotopic ossification. *Journal of Clinical Investigation*, *125*(8), 3117–3131. http://doi.org/10.1172/JCI80313

Zhang, J., He, F., Zhang, W., Zhang, M., Yang, H., & Luo, Z.-P. (2015). Mechanical force enhanced bony formation in defect implanted with calcium sulphate cement. *Bone Research*, *3*, 14048. http://doi.org/10.1038/boneres.2014.48

Zhao, Y., Paderu, P., Delmas, G., Dolgov, E., Lee, M. H., Senter, M. … Perlin, D. S. (2015). Carbohydrate-derived fulvic acid is a highly promising topical agent to enhance healing of wounds infected with drug-resistant pathogens. *The Journal of Trauma and Acute Care Surgery*, *79*(4 Suppl 2), S121–9. http://doi.org/10.1097/TA.0000000000000737

Zofková, I., Nemcikova, P., & Matucha, P. (2013). Trace elements and bone health. *Clinical Chemistry and Laboratory Medicine*, *51*(8), 1555–61. http://doi.org/10.1515/cclm-2012-0868

www.ingramcontent.com/pod-product-compliance
Lightning Source LLC
Chambersburg PA
CBHW070332190526
45169CB00005B/1851